# Progress in
# Medicinal Chemistry 40

# Progress in Medicinal Chemistry 40

*Series Editors:*

F.D. KING, B.SC., D.PHIL., C.CHEM., F.R.S.C.　and　A.W. OXFORD, M.A., D.PHIL.

*GlaxoSmithKline*
*New Frontiers Science Park (North)*
*Third Avenue*
*Harlow, Essex CM19 5AW*
*United Kingdom*

*Consultant in Medicinal*
*Chemistry*
*P.O. Box 151*
*Royston SG8 5YQ*
*United Kingdom*

*Guest Editors:*

ALLEN B. REITZ, PH.D.　and　SCOTT L. DAX, PH.D.

*Johnson & Johnson*
*Pharmaceutical R&D*
*Spring House, PA 19477-0766*
*USA*

*Johnson & Johnson*
*Pharmaceutical R&D*
*Spring House,*
*PA 19477-0766 USA*

*2002*

ELSEVIER
AMSTERDAM·LONDON·NEW YORK·OXFORD·PARIS·SHANNON·TOKYO

ELSEVIER SCIENCE B.V.
Sara Burgerhartstraat 25
P.O. Box 211, 1000 AE Amsterdam, The Netherlands

First edition 2002
Library of Congress Cataloging in Publication Data
A catalog record from the Library of Congress has been applied for.

ISBN:           0 444 51054 0
ISSN Series:    0079 6468

⊗  The paper used in this publication meets the requirements of ANSI/NISO Z39.48-1992 (Permanence of Paper). Printed in The Netherlands.

# Contents

# Preface

Medicinal Chemistry continues as an integral part of the Drug Discovery process, at the interface of classic organic synthesis and biology or pharmacology. It is one of the most rewarding and exciting areas of research, as the authors of the chapters in this special volume of *Progress in Medicinal Chemistry* would certainly attest. In this guest-edited volume four contributions are included describing medicinal chemistry research in action from the basic understanding of structure and function provided by computational methods and in vitro pharmacological proof-of-concept experiments, to (Structure-Activity Relationship) SAR development that has led to marketed therapeutic agents, or advanced clinical candidates.

Bob Hudkins and colleagues at Cephalon provide a thorough discussion of the development of CEP-1347, a potent inhibitor of the JNK kinase pathway, and a small-molecule that thwarts neurodegenerative processes in neurons, including programmed cell-death (apoptosis). The saga of CEP-1347 is rich in pharmacological studies that address issues of kinase selectivity and signal transduction, along with a diverse assortment of highly specialized cellular assays and animal models that elucidate efficacy against a battery of insult conditions. The research is aimed at providing a therapeutic strategy to treat Parkinson's Disease and potentially other such neurodegenerative conditions that are poorly managed using the pharmaceutical armament available today.

Dave Ferguson and colleagues at the Department of Medicinal Chemistry of the University of Minnesota describe modeling studies comparing the mu, delta, and kappa opioid receptors. Using the structure of the G-protein coupled receptor rhodopsin as a template, they have analyzed the opioid receptors in a way that provides insight as to the preferred modes of binding of small-molecule opioid ligands. This type of research in the future will enable medicinal chemists to design more potent and selective agents acting at the opioid receptors.

Jeffrey Corbett and Jim Rodgers (Dupont Pharmaceuticals) describe the development of a new generation of non-nucleoside reverse transcriptase inhibitors that originate from efavirenz, the first NNRTI approved by the

FDA as a first line therapy to treat HIV infection and AIDS. Their account details not only SAR optimization of the series but also addresses potency against mutant enzymes, cellular permeability and protein binding. This multi-faceted approach has led to several clinical candidates that offer superior anti-viral properties compared to efavirenz.

Bruce Roth from Pfizer provides a gripping account of the discovery and development of atorvastatin (LipitorR). Since it was potentially the fourth HMGCoA reductase inhibitor to be introduced, clinical evaluation of the compound required courage and commitment. The commercial success of atorvastatin has provided ample proof of the wisdom of the research and strategic approach that was taken.

January 2002                                            Scott L. Dax
                                                       Allen B. Reitz
                       Johnson & Johnson Pharmaceutical
                              Research and Development
                                        Guest Editors

# List of Contributors

**J.W. Corbett**
Dupont Pharmaceuticals Company, Experimental Station,
P.O. Box 80500, Wilmington, DE 19880-0500

**D.M. Ferguson**
Department of Medicinal Chemistry, University of Minnesota,
Minneapolis, MN 55455

**R.L. Hudkins**
Departments of Medicinal Chemistry and Neurobiology
Cephalon Inc., 145 Brandywine Parkway West Chester,
PA 19380, USA

**E. Jorvig**
Department of Medicinal Chemistry, University of Minnesota,
Minneapolis, MN 55455

**A.C. Maroney**
Departments of Medicinal Chemistry and Neurobiology
Cephalon Inc., 145 Brandywine Parkway West Chester,
PA 19380, USA

**I. McFadyen**
Department of Medicinal Chemistry, University of Minnesota,
Minneapolis, MN 55455

**T. Metzger**
Department of Medicinal Chemistry, University of Minnesota,
Minneapolis, MN 55455

**G. Poda**
Department of Medicinal Chemistry, University of Minnesota,
Minneapolis, MN 55455

**J.D. Rodgers**
Dupont Pharmaceuticals Company, Experimental Station,
P.O. Box 80500, Wilmington, DE 19880-0500

**B.D. Roth**
Department of Chemistry, Pfizer Global Research and
Development, Ann Arbor Laboratories, 2800 Plymouth Road,
Ann Arbor, MI 48170

**G. Subramanian**
Department of Medicinal Chemistry, University of Minnesota,
Minneapolis, MN 55455

**M.S. Saporito**
Departments of Medicinal Chemistry and Neurobiology
Cephalon Inc., 145 Brandywine Parkway West Chester,
PA 19380, USA

Progress in Medicinal Chemistry – Vol. 40,
Series Editors: F.D. King and A.W. Oxford
Guest Editors: A.B. Reitz and S.L. Dax
© 2002 Elsevier Science B.V. All rights reserved.

# 1 The Discovery and Development of Atorvastatin, a Potent Novel Hypolipidemic Agent

BRUCE D. ROTH*

*Department of Chemistry, Pfizer Global Research and Development, Ann Arbor Laboratories, 2800 Plymouth Road, Ann Arbor, MI 48170, U.S.A.*

ABSTRACT

The search for potent and efficacious inhibitors of the enzyme HMG-CoA reductase (HMGRI) was the focus of considerable research in the 1980s. Building on the discovery of the fungal metabolite-derived inhibitors, mevastatin, lovastatin, pravastatin and simvastatin, a number of totally synthetic inhibitors were discovered and developed. This manuscript describes the discovery and development of one of those synthetic inhibitors, atovastatin calcium, currently marketed in the United States as LIPITOR®. This inhibitor was designed based in part on molecular modeling comparisons of the structures of the fungal metabolites and other synthetically derived inhibitors. In addition to development of the structure-activity relationships which led to atorvastatin calcium, another critical aspect of the development of this area was the parallel improvement in the chemistry required to prepare compounds of the increased synthetic complexity needed to potently inhibit this enzyme. Ultimately, the development of several chiral syntheses of enantiomerically pure atorvastatin calcium was accomplished through a collaborative effort between discovery and development. The impact of the progress of the required chemistry as well as external factors on internal decision-making with regards to the development of atorvastatin calcium will be discussed.

*Tel (734) 622-7737; Fax (734) 622-3107

The biosynthesis of cholesterol from acetyl-CoA involves a process of more than 20 biosynthetic steps *(Figure 1.1)* [1]. This tightly controlled pathway is regulated by the levels of low-density lipoprotein (LDL)-receptors on liver cells as the means of ensuring whole-body cholesterol homeostasis [2]. It has been known since the late 1950's and early 1960's that inhibition of cholesterol biosynthesis was an effective means of lowering plasma cholesterol in both animals [3] and man [4]. What was unclear was whether it could be done safely. In fact there were many doubts based on the experience with the triparanol (MER-23, **1**, *Figure 1.2*) which caused cataracts in humans [5]. Despite this setback, the criteria for a safe and effective inhibitor of cholesterol bio-

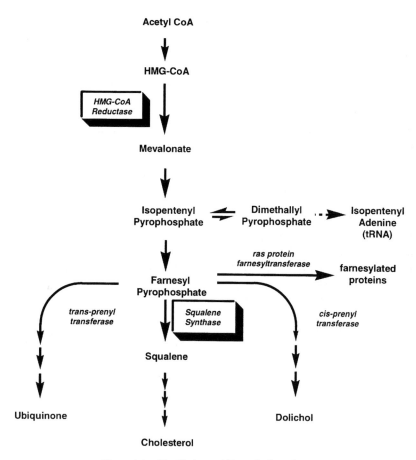

*Figure 1.1. The Cholesterol biosynthetic pathway.*

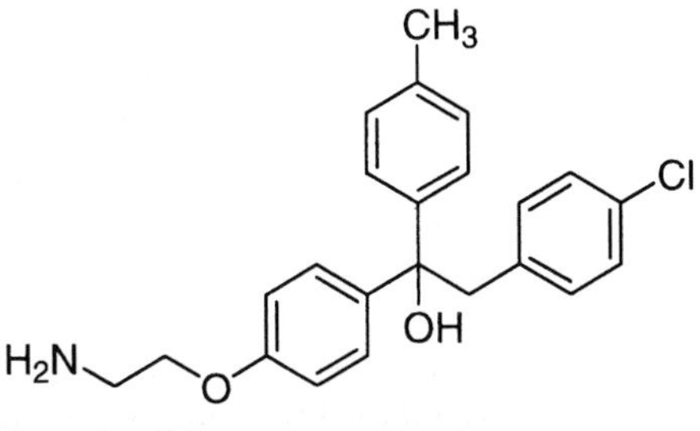

*Figure 1.2.   Triparanol (MER-29).*

synthesis were clearly articulated by Curran and Azarnoff in 1957 [6]. Their postulate was that safe inhibition could be achieved by blocking the pathway after the formation of acetoacetate, but prior to the formation of squalene. When in-depth mechanistic studies were performed with triparanol, not surprisingly, it was discovered that it broke this rule by inhibiting the pathway at the pentultimate step in the biosynthetic pathway, as evidenced by the accumulation of desmosterol in the plasma and tissues of patients treated with this drug [7]. Further studies demonstrated that it was also desmosterol which accumulated in the lens of patients [8], emphasizing the potential dangers of inhibiting steps late in the biosynthetic pathway and causing medical concerns that would follow this area of research for decades. In fact, as recently as 1992, there were calls for a moratorium on the use of cholesterol-lowering drugs in primary prevention of myocardial infarction (MI) due to the lack of data from long-term clinical trials demonstrating a reduction not just in cardiovascular mortality, but in total mortality as well [9]. This concern was not completely alleviated until the results of the Scandinavian Simvastatin Survival Study were published in 1994 demonstrating reductions in total mortality with long-term statin treatment [10].

Despite the findings with triparanol, the search for cholesterol biosynthesis inhibitors continued unabated fueled by the hope that inhibition pre-squalene would avoid the formation of non-metabolizable sterol intermediates, such as desmosterol, and result in a safe and effect treatment for hypercholesterolemia [11].

The enzyme which became the focus of attention in the search for cholesterol biosynthesis inhibitors was 3-hydroxy-3-methylglutaryl-coenzyme A reductase (HMGR, EC 1.1.1.34), the rate-limiting and first committed step in the biosynthetic pathway. This membrane-bound, endoplasmic reticulum localized enzyme catalyzes the two-step conversion of (S)-3-hydroxy-3-methylglutaryl-coenzyme A to 3-(R)-mevalonic acid through a putative hemi-thioacetal (*Figure 1.3*) [12]. Given that this hemi-thioacetal most likely represents a

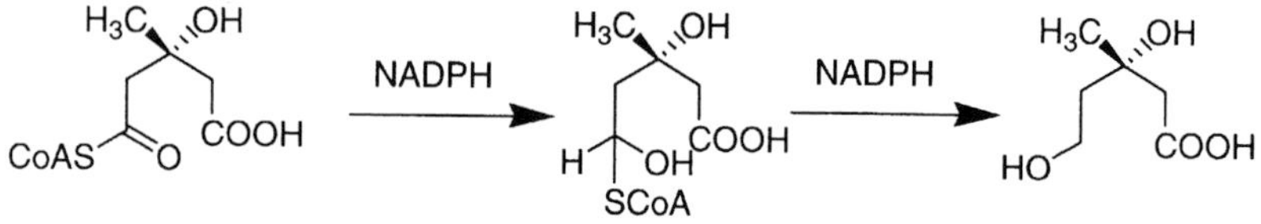

*Figure 1.3.  Reduction of HMG-CoA catalyzed by HMGR.*

transition-state intermediate, it should not have been surprising when screening of fermentation beers resulted in the isolation of compounds that closely mimicked this structure.

The first fermentation product identified was isolated almost simultaneously by two separate laboratories and given the name compactin (later changed to mevastatin) by the Beecham group, who isolated it as an antifungal from strains of the microorganism *Penicillium brevicompactum* and determined its molecular structure by x-ray crystallography (**2**, *Figure 1.4*) [13]. The second group, from the Fermentation Research Laboratories at Sankyo, isolated the identical compound from cultures of *Penicillium citrinum*, but discovered it was a potent and competitive inhibitor of rat liver HMGR in vitro and sterol synthesis in vivo and gave it the code number ML-236B [14]. Further studies with ML-236B demonstrated that it decreased serum total and LDL-cholesterol in dogs [15], monkeys [16], and human patients with heterozygous familial hypercholesterolemia [17]. Shortly after the discovery of compactin, a second fungal metabolite (**3**), differing from compactin by a single methyl group was isolated from cultures of *Aspergillus terreus* by workers at Merck [18] (and named mevinolin) and from *Monascus ruber* by the Sankyo group (and named Monacolin K) [19]. This compound was found to inhibit rat liver HMGR twice as potently as compactin (Ki of 0.6 nM vs 1.4 nM) [18] and was later renamed lovastatin. Ultimately, **3** would be the first HMGR inhibitor (HMGRI) approved by the U.S. Food and Drug Administration for the treatment of hypercholesterolemia and would be marketed by Merck Sharpe and Dohme under the trade name Mevacor®. Two other potent fungal metabolite HMGRIs would ultimately become marketed drugs, pravastatin (**4**), produced by microbial hydroxylation of compactin [20] and simvastatin (**5**) produced by synthetic modification of lovastatin [21]. Although all of these compounds were potent HMGR inhibitors and effective cholesterol-lowering agents, in the early 1980's concern over the viability of these compounds was created by the termination of the development of compactin in 1980 due to safety concerns created by results from preclinical toxicology experiments [22]. This apparently also led to a temporary suspension of the development of lovastatin. Thus, even though the fungal metabolites as a class would ultimately prove extremely safe and effective in clinical trials, in the early 1980's there was at least a perceived need

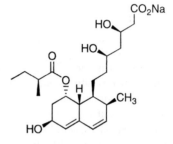

2, compactin (mevastatin)

3, lovastatin (MEVACOR®)

4, simvastatin (ZOCOR®)

5, pravastatin (PRAVACOL®)

*Figure 1.4. Fungal metabolite inhibitors of HMGR.*

for structurally novel HMGR inhibitors such that any non-mechanism related toxicity would be avoided.

The first indication that the complex hexahydronaphthalene portion of the fungal metabolites could be replaced with a simpler ring system without loss of biological activity appeared in a patent application [23], then in publication form, from the Merck, Sharpe and Dohme Research Labs [24]. In this disclosure, it was revealed that ortho-biphenyl containing 3,5-dihydroxy-6-heptenoic acids and their lactones, such as 6 (*Figure 1.5*), were equipotent to the fungal metabolites at inhibiting HMGR in vitro. This disclosure led us to develop the hypothesis that the key requirements for potent inhibition of HMGR were a mevalonolactone/3,5-dihydroxy-heptanoic or -6-heptenoic acid moiety and a large lipophilic group held in the correct spatial relationship by a spacer or template group [25]. If this were true, then virtually any ring system which fulfilled this requirement would lead to a series of potent inhibitors. This hypothesis was apparently shared by other laboratories and a large number of

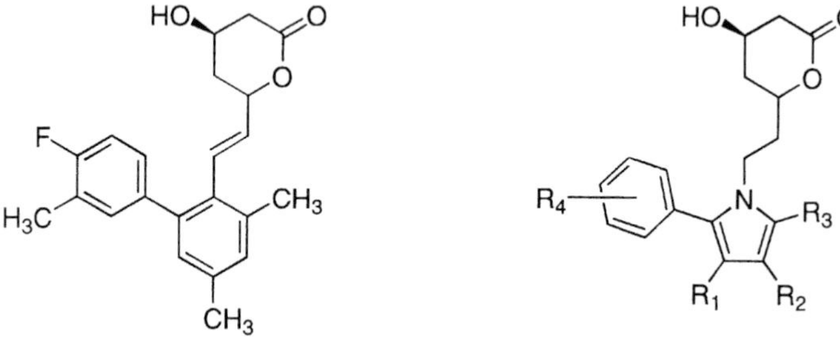

6

Pyrrole Template

*Figure 1.5. HMGR inhibitor templates.*

diverse series of inhibitors were discovered and developed based on this model [26].

We selected the 1H-pyrrole ring system as our starting template to test this hypothesis, primarily because these could readily be prepared from 1,4-dike-tones through the classical Paal-Knorr condensation [27] (see retrosynthesis in *Scheme 1.1*) and these 1,4-diketones, in turn, were potentially available pos-sessing a wide variety of 1- and 4-substituents employing the thiazolium salt chemistry developed by Stetter [28].

In practice, this scheme proved highly effective and a large number of 1,2,5-trisubstituted pyrroles were prepared using several omega-aminopropionitriles as the amine component to introduce a latent aldehyde. Unveiling of these latent aldehydes by DIBAL reduction followed by condensation with the dia-nion of methyl or ethyl acetoacetate employing the procedure of Weiler [29] introduced the remaining carbons needed in the targeted compounds. Un-fortunately, though expedient, this chemistry introduced the 5-hydroxyl as a racemic mixture, a problem that would need to be corrected later. Despite this less than optimal solution to the stereochemical requirements at C-5, we were able to control the relative configurations of the 3- and 5-hydroxyls by appli-cation of the predominantly syn-selective reduction of β-hydroxy ketones de-veloped by Narasaka and Pai [30]. In general, this protocol afforded approximately a 10:1 ratio of syn/anti diastereomers. Lactonization by reflux in toluene produced the corresponding lactones from which the cis-diastereomer could be removed by recrystallization. The pure trans-diastereomers were then ring-opened by base hydrolysis to provide the biologically active dihydroxy-acids. This general synthesis is illustrated by the synthesis of the 2-(4-fluoro-phenyl)-5-isopropyl analog (**12**) shown in *Scheme 1.2*.

The initial question addressed was determination of the optimal spacing between the mevalonolactone and the pyrrole ring. This was rapidly narrowed

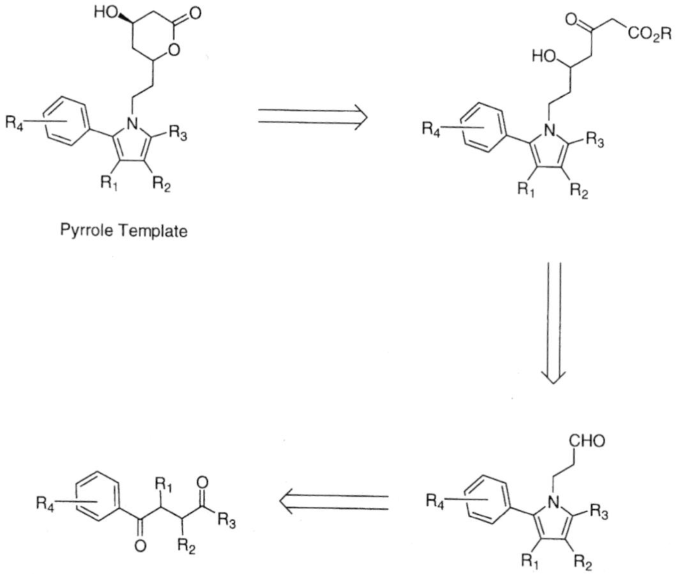

Scheme 1.1. *Pyrrole inhibitor retrosynthesis.*

to a two-atom linker through the synthesis of a small group of analogs (*Table 1.1*).

With this established, we next prepared a series of approximately thirty 2,5-disubstituted analogs possessing a range of substituted aromatic, cyclic, branched and straight-chain aliphatic groups to define the optimal substituents at the 2- and 5-positions. The conclusion from this exercise was that the distance across the pyrrole ring from the tip of the 2-substituent to the tip of the 5-substituent could be no longer than 10 angstroms with the size of the 2-substituent being no more than 5.9 angstroms and the 5-substituent being no more than 3.3 angstroms. Further refinement of this analysis revealed that best potency was contained in compound **12** possessing a 4-fluorophenyl in the 2-position and an isopropyl in the 5-position of the pyrrole ring [25].Unfortunately, this compound still possessed only one-tenth of the inhibitory potency of mevastatin (*Table 1.2*). Taking into account the likely scenario that all of the biological activity was contained in one stereoisomer, we were still considerably short of the target potency and had come to the limit of what could be accomplished using the current synthetic route. In these circumstances, the options are to find alternate series or to attempt to ascertain the source of the deficiency. To this end, a simple molecular modeling exercise was undertaken to compare the differences between our best compound and those reported by

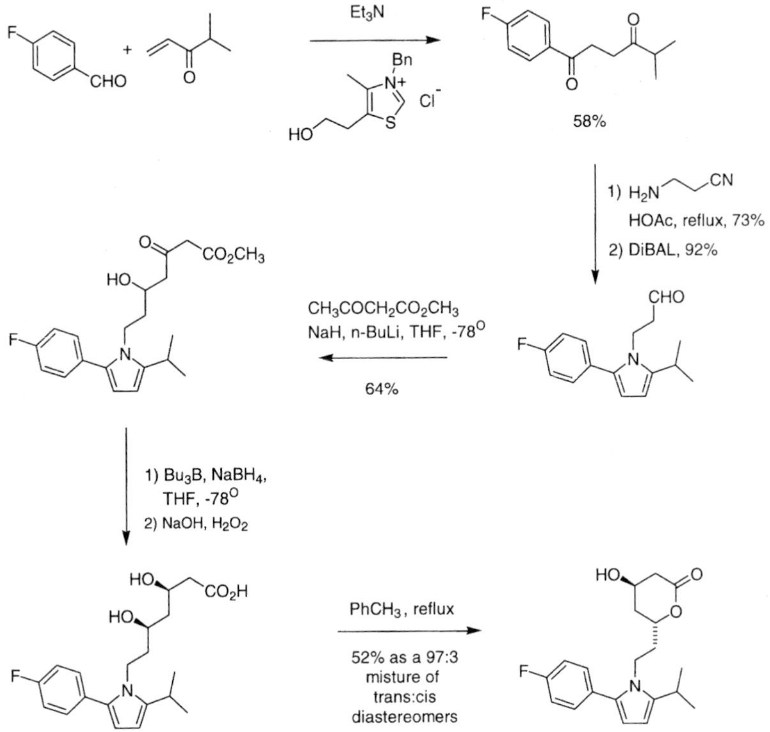

Scheme 1.2.  Synthesis of 1,2,5-trisubstituted pyrrole inhibitors.

Merck. The simple overlay of these molecules (see *Figure 1.6*) revealed the presence of a methyl group in the Merck compound in a region of space not occupied by our inhibitors.

To determine the importance of occupying this space, bromine and chlorines were introduced into the 3- and 4-positions of our most potent analog (**12**) employing the synthetic route described in *Scheme 1.3* [31]. After testing the ability of these compounds to inhibit rat-liver HMGR, we were gratified to find that both compounds possessed inhibitory potencies comparable to the fungal metabolites (*Table 1.3*).

Although initially we were excited by this finding, the 3,4-dibromo analog **19** was taken into early preclinical development and rapidly found to display considerable toxicity [32]. As it turned out, much of the toxicology had been observed by others and was found to be specific to rodents or was derived from exaggerated pharmacology at high dosage levels and was most

Table 1.1.  OPTIMIZATION OF THE LINKER GROUP

| Compound No. | X | $IC_{50}(\mu M)^a$ |
|---|---|---|
| 7 | | 20 |
| 8 | | 24 |
| 9 | | >100 |
| 10 | -CH₂CH₂CH₂- | 53 |
| 11 | -CH₂CH₂- | 0.5 |

[a] Inhibition of[14C]-acetate conversion to cholesterol employing crude rat liver homogenate (ref. 24).

Table 1.2.  VARIATION AT THE PYRROLE 5-POSITION

| Compound No. | R | $IC_{50}(\mu M)^a$ |
|---|---|---|
| 11 | -CH₃ | 0.57 |
| 12 | -CH(CH₃)₂ | 0.40 |
| 13 | -C(CH₃)₃ | 1.6 |
| 14 | -CH(CH₂CH₃)₂ | 20 |
| 15 | -Cyclopropyl | 2.2 |
| 16 | -Cyclobutyl | 17 |
| 17 | -Cyclohexyl | >100 |

[a] Inhibition of [14C]-acetate conversion to cholesterol using a crude rat liver homogenate. Mevastatin $IC_{50} = 0.026\,\mu M$ (ref. 24).

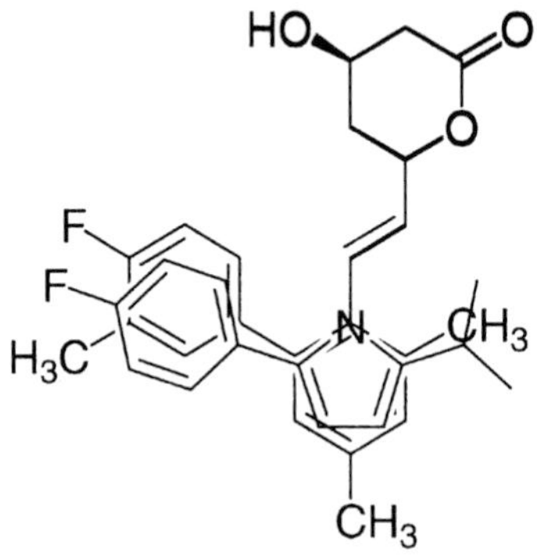

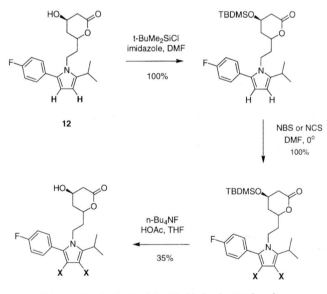

*Figure 1.6   Overlay of HMGR inhibitor templates.*

severe with very bioavailable inhibitors which achieved high plasma and tissue concentrations [33,34]. Once again, we were faced with a decision point in the pyrrole series. Since we did not know whether the toxicity observed was related to the mechanism of action, the pyrrole series or the presence of the bromines in the 3- and 4-positions, rather than abandoning

*Scheme 1.3.   Synthesis of the 3,4-dihalosubstituted analogs.*

Table 1.3.  EFFECT OF HALOGEN SUBSTITUTION, AT THE PYRROLE
3- AND 4-POSITIONS

| Compound No. | X | $IC_{50}(\mu M)^a$ |
|---|---|---|
| 12 | H | 0.23 |
| 18 | Cl | 0.028 |
| 19 | Br | 0.028 |
| 2 (mevastatin) | | 0.030 |

[a]Inhibition of the conversion of D, L-[$^{14}$C]-HMG-CoA to mevalonic acid using partially purified rat liver HMGR (ref. 30).

the pyrrole series, a two-pronged approach was taken of both looking for alternative series [35,36] and synthesizing 3,4-non-halogen-substituted pyrroles in the hope that these compounds would retain activity, but lack toxicity. Unfortunately, the requirement for a penta-substituted pyrrole also required the development of an entirely new synthetic route to effectively develop the SAR at the 3- and 4-positions, since the existing route was limited only to those substituents that could be introduced by electrophilic substitution. A possible solution was presented through the 3 + 2 cycloaddition of azlactones and acetylenes pioneered by Huisgen [37]. This chemistry proved to be a very versatile means of preparing pentasubstituted pyrroles from α-amidoacids and acetylenes containing at least one electron withdrawing group (esters, nitriles, carboxamides) [31]. Although yields were best with acetylenes containing two electron withdrawing groups (e.g., dimethylacetylene dicarboxylate), acceptable yields could be obtained with those possessing only one electron withdrawing group (40–60%). As significant, in the case of the unsymmetrical phenylacetylenes, considerable regiocontrol over the orientation of the 3- and 4-substituents could be achieved by adjustment of the substituents derived from the amide and amino acid precursors (*Scheme 1.4*). Using this methodology, followed by application of the Weiler dianion chemistry and stereoselective reduction used previously, a series of compounds were made with the already optimized 2-(4-fluorophenyl) and 5-isopropyl substitution and a variety of phenyl, substituted phenyl, ester, amide and nitriles at the 3- and 4-positions (*Table 1.4*).

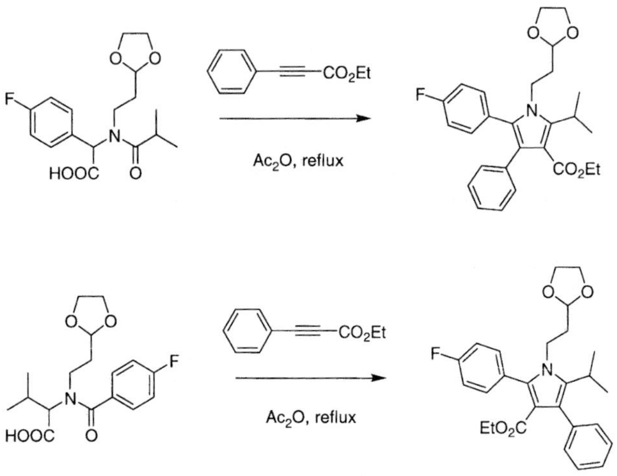

Scheme 1.4.  Regiocontrol in 3 + 2 cycloaddition mediated pyrrole synthesis.

Table 1.4.  SUMMARY OF 2-(4-FLUOROPHENYL)-5-ISOPROPYL-3,4-DISUBSTITUTED
PYRROLES

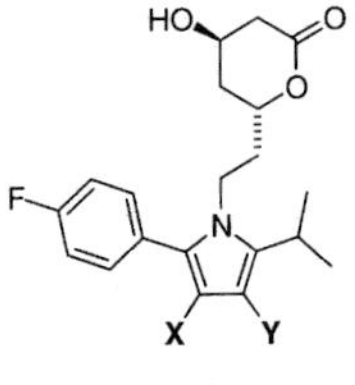

| Compound No | X | Y | $IC_{50}(\mu M)^a$ |
|---|---|---|---|
| 20 | $CO_2Me$ | $CO_2Me$ | 0.18 |
| 21 | $CO_2Et$ | $CO_2Et$ | 0.35 |
| 22 | Ph | $CO_2Et$ | 0.17 |
| 23 | $CO_2Et$ | Ph | 0.050 |
| 24 | Ph | $CO_2CH_2Ph$ | 0.040 |
| 24 | Ph | CONHPh | 0.025 |
| ( + )- 24 | Ph | CONHPh | $0.007^b$ |
| (−)- 24 | Ph | CONHPh | $0.44^c$ |
| 2(mevastatin) | | | 0.030 |

[a] Inhibition of conversion of D,L -[$^{14}$C]-HMG-CoA to mevalonic acid using partially purified rat crude liver HMGR (ref. 30).
[b] Contaminated with 3% of (−)-24.
[c] Contaminated with 3% of ( + )-24.

1,2,3,5-Tetrasubstituted analogs were available by application of the Stetter chemistry to substituted cinnamoylesters followed by decarboxylation (*Scheme 1.5*).

Due to the difficulty in synthesis, a total of only 20 analogs were prepared, with best activity found in the 3-phenyl, 4-carboxamidophenyl analog (**24**). Separation of the two enantiomers of **24** by synthesis and separation of the diastereomeric *R*-α-methylbenzylamides followed by hydrolysis demonstrated that, as expected, all of the biological activity resided in one stereoisomer, ( + )-**24**. This isomer was later confirmed to be the *R,R*-stereoisomer by total synthesis [31] and x-ray crystallography and found to possess inhibitory potency approaching that of simvastatin in vitro. Scale-up of this analog and preliminary testing in vivo in both casein-fed rabbit and cholestyramine-primed dog models of hypercholesterolemia demonstrated that ( + )-**24** possessed potency and efficacy in vivo comparable to that found with lovastatin (unpublished data). In subsequent studies done under more carefully controlled conditions with larger groups of animals, it was determined that atorvastatin was actually more potent and efficacious than lovastatin at lowering LDL-cholesterol in rabbits [38] and guinea pigs [39] and triglycerides in rats [39].

Having identified a potent and efficacious HMGR inhibitor, we were now faced with a critical decision, that of whether to develop our compound as the racemate or the pure stereoisomer. In fact, Sandoz when faced with this de-

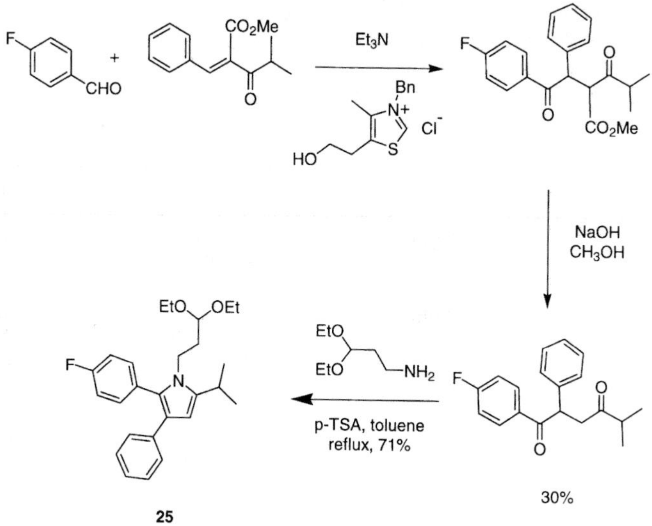

**25**

*Scheme 1.5. Synthesis of 1,2,3,5-tetra substituted pyrroles.*

cision in the development of fluvastatin chose to develop it as the racemate [26]. We chose to develop atorvastatin as the pure stereoisomer, for several reasons: 1) to avoid the unnecessary burden to the patient of having to metabolize 50% of possibly inert material (the wrong enantiomer) and 2) the desire to avoid having an obvious disadvantage (potency) in a compound entering the marketplace potentially 10 years after the fungal metabolite-derived inhibitors.

Having made this decision, we formed two teams of chemists working in parallel towards a chiral synthesis, one in Discovery Chemistry in Ann Arbor and a second in Chemical Development in Holland, Michigan. The first challenge was actually not the chiral synthesis, but scaling the achiral parts of the existing process that would be needed for the ultimate chiral synthesis. One of the initial problems was scaling the $3 + 2$ cycloaddition reaction used previously, in that, excess phenylamidocarbonyl phenylacetylene was required to achieve good yields, but this proved very difficult to separate from the product on large scale. Conceptually, the solution could be derived from the Paal-Knorr cyclization, if an appropriate amine would cyclodehydrate with the properly substituted 1,4-diketone. This route would also open up the possibility of a convergent synthesis employing a fully elaborated side-chain ( *Scheme 1.6*).

We therefore set about the preparation of the requisite 1,4-diketone using the Stetter methodology. However, we were disappointed to find that we were unable to achieve the desired cyclodehydration under a variety of conditions (*Scheme 1.6*). Fortunately, the Holland group had better success with this transformation (vide infra).

Because of our inability to affect the Paal-Knorr condensation with the fully substituted diketone, as an alternative, we examined the synthesis of the tetra-substituted pyrrole **25** (*Scheme 1.7*) based on the assumption that the carbox-amide could be introduced later in the sequence. In the event, Paal-Knorr cyclization of the less highly substituted diketone proceeded smoothly to produce **25** in modest yield (*Scheme 1.11*). Subsequent introduction of the N-phenyl carboxamide proceeded smoothly by bromination with N-bromo-succinimide, followed by lithium halogen exchange and reaction of the re-sultant heteroaryl lithium with phenyl isocyanate. Hydrolysis then afforded the aldehyde **26** prepared previously employing the $3 + 2$ cycloaddition protocol [31]. All of these transformations were scalable and proceeded in acceptable yield. Our strategy in Ann Arbor for introducing the 5-R-hydroxyl involved application of the diastereoselective aldol condensation of Braun [40] to al-dehyde **26** (*Scheme 1.13*). Thus, condensation of **26** with the magnesium dia-nion of S-( + )-2-acetoxy-1,1,2-triphenylethanol afforded a 96:4 ratio of the S,R and S,S-diastereomers in 60% yield. This ratio could be improved to 98:2 with one recrystallization [31]. Ester exchange with sodium methoxide followed by reaction with excess lithio-*t*-butylacetate afforded the R-δ-hydroxy-β-ketoester made previously as the racemate. Reduction with $Bu_3B$-$NaBH_4$ as before the

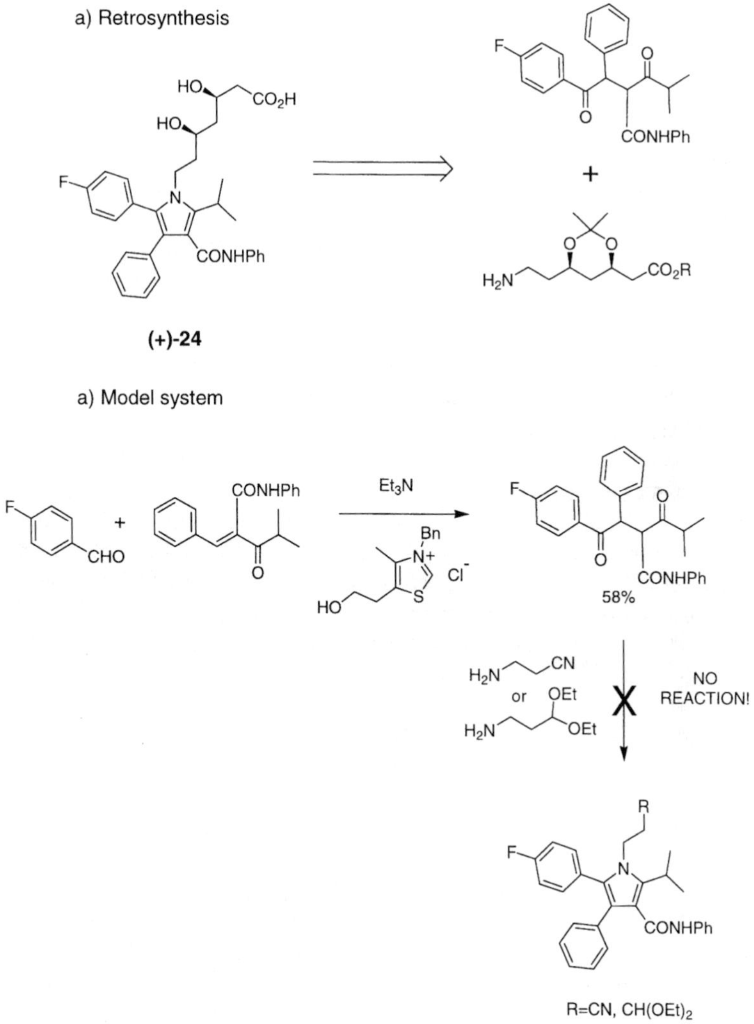

a) Retrosynthesis

(+)-24

a) Model system

R=CN, CH(OEt)$_2$

*Scheme 1.6. Optimal retrosynthesis of (+)-24 and failed model study.*

afforded the syn-β,δ-dihydroxyester which after hydrolysis, acidification and lactonization afforded crude lactone (+)-24. Fortuitously, the *d,l*-pair crystallized out of ethyl acetate-hexanes and 100% enatiomerically pure (+)-24 could be isolated from the mother liquors.

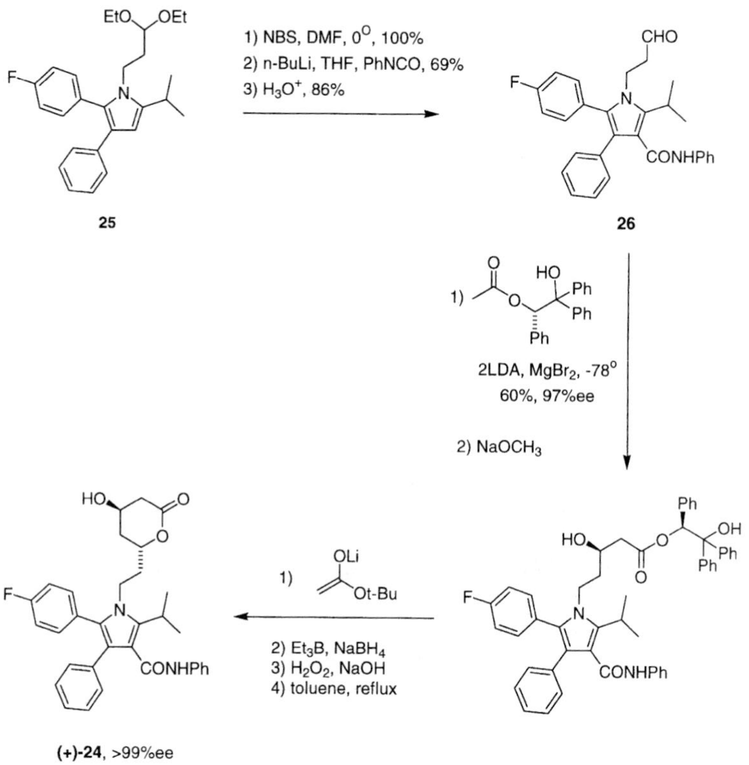

Scheme 1.7.   Synthesis of ( + )-**24**.

Although this route was successful in producing gram quantities of enantiomerically pure ( + )-**24**, because of the linear nature of this route, the number of low-temperature reactions involved and the relatively low yields in some of the final steps such as the final purification, its potential for scale-up to provide the kilogram quantities needed for further development was low. Thus, for the synthesis to be economically viable, the Holland group was forced to develop an entirely different approach [41,42]. A critical component of this effort was an extensive investigation of the Paal-Knorr conducted by Alan Millar in Chemical Development which finally resulted in a successful cyclodehydration in the model system when a full equivalent of pivalic acid was used as catalyst (*Scheme 1.8*). This afforded pentasubstitued pyrrole **27** in 43% yield and demonstrated that a totally convergent synthesis was possible. This now became the ultimate goal.

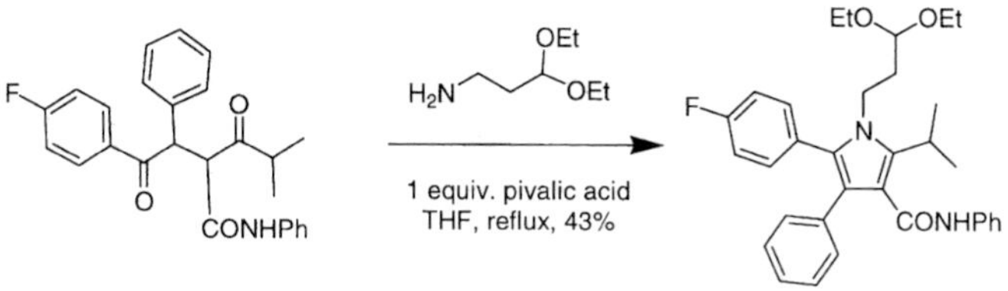

**Scheme 1.8.** *Paal-Knorr synthesis of pentasubstituted pyrroles.*

To this end, several routes passing through the known (*S*)-methyl-4-bromo-3-hydroxybutyrate **28**, an intermediate used in prior syntheses of HMGRIs [43], were developed [41]. This key intermediate was derived most efficiently from isoascorbic acid as has been reported previously [43–45], such that it was produced as a single stereoisomer (*Scheme 1.9*). Protection of **28** as the *t*-butyl-dimethylsilylether [43], followed by conversion to the nitrile provided an advanced intermediate (**29**) that could be taken in several directions.

Thus, **29** could be hydrolyzed to the acid and chain extended by activation with *N,N*-carbonyldiimidazole followed by reaction with the magnesium salt of potassium *t*-butyl malonate [46]. Acidification followed by deprotection with buffered fluoride afforded the δ-hydroxy-β-ketoester **30** which was converted to the syn-1,3-diol employing $NaBH_4$ and $Et_2BOMe$, a slight modification of the original procedure [47]. Protection of the diol as the acetonide produced the nicely crystalline nitrile **31** in 65% yield and with diastereoselectivity in the range of 100:1. One recrystallization improved this ratio to >350:1. Reduction of the nitrile with molybdenum-doped Raney-Nickel catalyst then afforded the desired side-chain (**32**) with outstanding enantiomeric excess (>99.5) (*Scheme 1.10*) [41].

An alternate, shorter route involved reaction of the alcohol derived from **29** with 3–4 equivalents of lithium tert-butyl acetate to afford an excellent 75–80% yield of hydroxyketone **30** without the need for prior protection of the alcohol and with no detectable reaction with the nitrile (*Scheme 1.11*). Although these routes still involved a low-temperature reduction, both could still be scaled to kilogram quantities [41].

Cyclization of the fully functionalized, stereochemically pure side-chain **32** with the fully substituted diketone under carefully defined conditions (1 eq. pivalic acid, 1:4:1 toluene-heptane-THF, *Scheme 1.12*) then afforded a 75% yield of pyrrole **33**. Deprotection and formation of the hemi-calcium salt produced stereochemically pure atorvastatin calcium in a convergent, commercially viable manner which accomplished the original vision for the

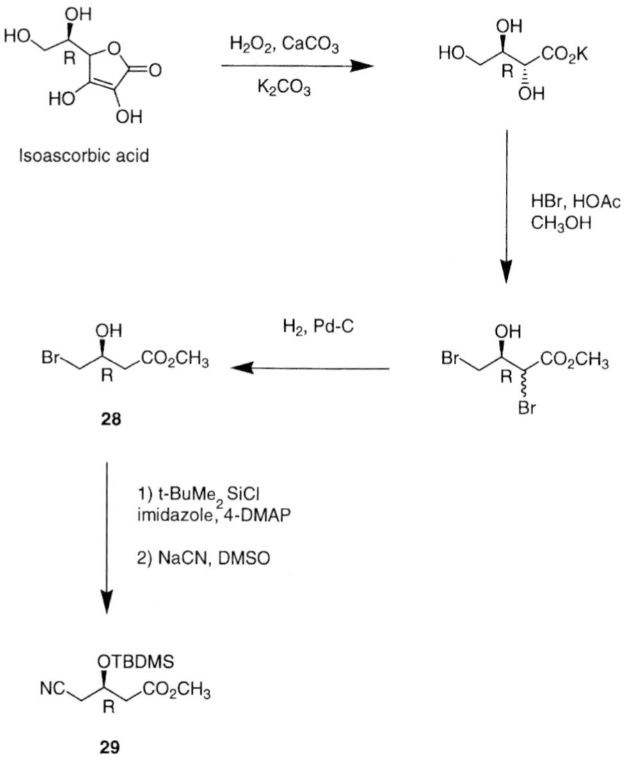

Scheme 1.9. *Synthesis of (S)-methyl-4-bromo-3-hydroxybutyrate* **28**.

synthesis developed in discovery chemistry, but was reduced to practice in chemical development.

Although one might have expected that the decision to take atorvastatin calcium into clinical development would be straight-forward, it was not. By the time we completed the preclinical studies needed to file an Investigational New Drug Application (IND) with the Food and Drug Administration (FDA) in late 1989, Mevacor[R], Zocor[R], and Pravacol[R] had all been approved for marketing by the FDA. Thus, we were faced with the expectation of coming into the marketplace nearly a decade after at least three HMGRIs and possibly more (Lescol[R] was approved several years later by the FDA). Fortunately, by this time, evidence from preclinical efficacy studies was beginning to emerge suggesting that atorvastatin calcium may be more potent and efficacious than the fungal metabolite derived inhibitors at lowering total and LDL-cholesterol, at least in some animal models [38,39]. Encouraged by this positive data and

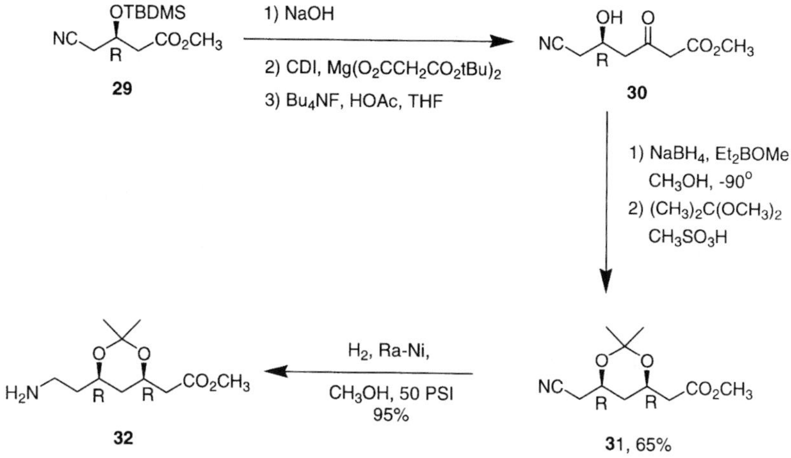

*Scheme 1.10.   Chiral side-chain synthesis.*

now having a scaleable process for synthesis of enantiomerically pure drug substance, the decision was taken by Dr. Ronnie Cresswell, then President of Parke-Davis Research, to move atorvastatin calcium into clinical trials in the hope that an improved efficacy profile would be observed in man over the then marketed drugs. To the delight of all those involved in the discovery and development of atorvastatin calcium, the merits of the drug were rapidly demonstrated in the phase 1 clinical trials in healthy volunteers where reductions in LDL-C approaching 60% were observed at the high dose of 80 mg/day (*Table 1.5*) [48]. This data provided the impetus for further development, since this level of efficacy was not achievable with other HMGRIs at approved doses or, in fact, with any other cholesterol-lowering drug. Since that original study in healthy volunteers, the outstanding potency and efficacy at lowering total cholesterol, LDL-cholesterol [49] and triglycerides [50] of atorvastatin calcium, now marketed in the United States as Lipitor®, has been reproduced and confirmed in numerous clinical studies and in many thousands of patients [51,52]. Today it has brought benefit to millions of patients and is one of the most widely prescribed pharmaceuticals in the world.

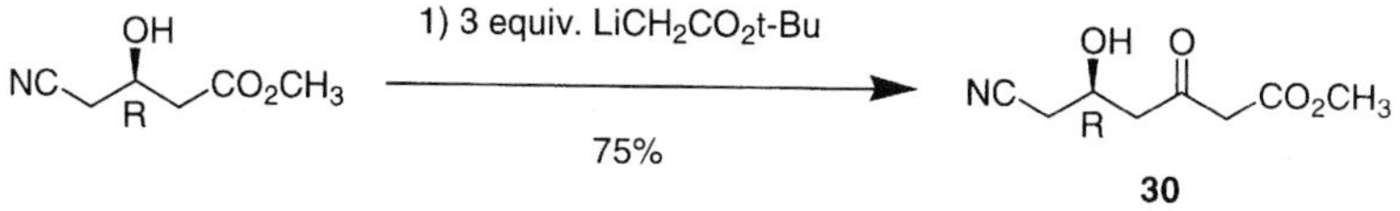

*Scheme 1.11.   Alternate chiral side-chain synthesis.*

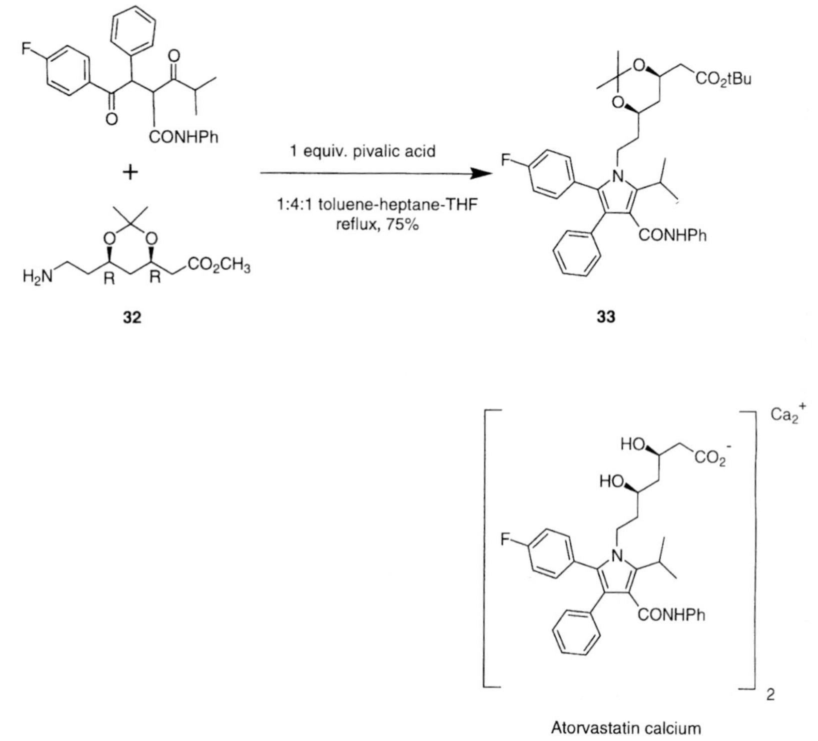
CONHPh
+
$H_2N$
R
R
$CO_2CH_3$
32
1 equiv. pivalic acid
1:4:1 toluene-heptane-THF
reflux, 75%
$CO_2tBu$
CONHPh
33
$Ca_2^+$
HO
HO
$CO_2^-$
CONHPh
2
Atorvastatin calcium

*Scheme 1.12. Convergent, chiral synthesis of atorvastation calcium.*

Table 1.5. MULTIPLE-DOSE TOLERANCE AND PHARMACOLOGIC EFFECT OF ATORVASTATIN CALCIUM IN HEALTHY VOLUNTEERS (REF. 48)

| *Dose (mg/d)* | *% change (mg/dL), Total Cholesterol* | *% change (mg/dL) LDL-Cholesterol* | *% change (mg/dL) Triglycerides* |
|---|---|---|---|
| Placebo | −3 | −3 | −3 |
| 10 | −22 | −31 | −12 |
| 20 | −30 | −39 | −30 |
| 40 | −36 | −47 | 0 |
| 80 | −45 | −58 | −22 |

# REFERENCES

1   Bloch, K. *Science* **1965**, *150(692)*, 19–28.
2   Goldstein, J. L., Brown, M. S. *J. Lipid Res.* **1984**, *25*, 1450–61
3   Blohm, T. R., MacKenzie, R. D. *Arch. Biochem. Biophys.* **1959**, *85*, 245.
4   Avigan, J., Steinberg, D., Vroman, H. E., Thompson, M. J., Mosettig, E. *J. Biol. Chem.* **1960**, *235*, 3123–3126.
5   Laughlin, R. C., Carey, T. F. *J. Amer. Med. Assoc.* **1962**, *181*, 339340.
6   Curran, G. L., Azarnoff, D. L. *Arch. Internal Med.* **1958**, *101*, 685–689.
7   Steinberg, D., Avigan, J. *J. Biol. Chem.* **1960**, *235*, 3127–3129.
8   Avigan, J., Steinberg, D., Thompson, M. J., Mossettig, E. *Biochem. Biophys. Res. Commun.* **1960**, *2*, 63–65.
9   Davey-Smith, G., Pekkanen, J. *BMJ* **1992**, *304*, 431–434.
10  Scandinavian Simvastatin Survival Study Group. *Lancet* **1994**, *344*, 1383–1389.
11  Boots, M. R., Boots, S. G., Noble, C. M., Guyer, K. E. *J. Pharm. Sci.* **1973**, *62*, 952.
12  Rogers, D. H., Panini, S. R., Rudney, H. *3-Hydroxy-3-methylglutaryl Coenzyme A Reductase;* Sabine, J. R., Ed.; CRC Press: Boca Raton, FL, 1983, Chapter 6, p. 66.
13  Brown, A. G., Smale, T. C., King, T. J., Hasenkamp, R., Thompson, R. H. *J. Chem. Soc. Perkin I* **1976**, 1165–1170.
14  Endo, A., Tsujita, Y., Kuroda, M., Tanzawa, K. *Eur. J. Biochem.* **1977**, *77*, 31–36.
15  Tsujita, Y., Kuroda, M., Tanzawa, K., Kitano, N., Endo, A. *Atherosclerosis* **1979**, *32*, 307–313.
16  Kuroda, M., Tsujita, Y., Tanzawa, K., Endo, A. *Lipids* **1979**, *14*, 858–589.
17  Mabuchi, H., Haba, T., Tatami, R., Miyamoto, S., Sakai, Y., Wakasugi, T., Watanabe, A., Koizumi, J., Takeda, R. *N. Engl. J. Med.* **1981**, *305*, 478–482.
18  Alberts, A. W., Chen, J., Kuron, G., Hunt, V., Huff, J., Hoffman, C., Rothrock, J., Lopez, M., Joshua, H., Harris, E., Patchett, A., Monaghan, R., Currie, S., Stapley, E., Albers-Schonberg, G., Hensens, O., Hirshfield, J., Hoogsteen, K., Liesch, J., Springer, J. *Proc. Nat. Acad. Sci. USA* **1980**, *77*, 3957–3961.
19  Endo, A. *J. Antibiotics* **1979**, *32*, 852–854.
20  Serizawa, N., Nakagawa, K., Hamano, K., Tsujita, Y., Terahara, A., Kuwano, H. *J. Antibiotics* **1983**, *36*, 604–607.
21  Hoffman, W. F., Alberts, A. W., Anderson, P. S., Chen, J. S., Smith, R. L., Willard, A. K. *J. Med. Chem.* **1986**, *29*, 849–852.
22  Endo, A. *Klin. Wochenschr.* **1988**, *66*, 421–427.
23  Willard, A. K., Novello, F. C., Hoffmann, W. F., Cragoe, E. J. Jr. *USP 4459422.*
24  Stokker, G. E., Alberts, A. W., Anderson, P. S., Cragoe, E. J. Jr., Deana, A. A., Gilfillan, J. L., Hirshfield, J., Holtz, W. J., Hoffman, W. F., et al. *J. Med. Chem.* **1986**, *29*, 170–181.
25  Roth, B. D., Ortwine, D. F., Hoefle, M. L., Stratton, C. D., Sliskovic, D. R., Wilson, M. W., Newton, R. S. *J. Med. Chem.* **1990**, *33*, 21–31.
26  Kathawala, F. G. *Trends in Medicinal Chemistry '88,* **1989**, 709–728.
27  Knorr, L. *Ber.* **1885**, *18*, 299; Paal, C. *Ber.* **1885**, *18*, 367.
28  Stetter, H. *Angew. Chem., Int. Ed. Eng.* **1976**, *15*, 639.
29  Huckin, S. N., Weiler, L. *J. Am. Chem. Soc.* **1981**, *103*, 6538–6539.
30  Narasaka, K., Pai, H. C. *Chem. Lett.* **1980**, 1415–1418.
31  Roth, B. D., Blankley, C. J., Chucholowski, A. W., Ferguson, E., Hoefle, M. L., Ortwine, D. F., Newton, R. S., Sekerke, C. S., Sliskovic, D. R., Stratton, C. D., Wilson, M.W. *J. Med. Chem.* **1991**, *34*, 357–366.
32  Sigler, R. E., Dominick, M. A., McGuire, E. J. *Toxicol. Pathol.* **1992**, *20*, 595–602.
33  MacDonald, J. S., Gerson, R. J., Kornbrust, D. J., Kloss, M. W., Prahalada, S., Berry, P. H., Alberts, A. W., Bokelman, D. L. *Am. J. Cardiol.* **1988**, *62*, 16J–27J.

34 Gerson, R. J., Allen, H. L., Lankas, G. R., MacDonald, J. S., Alberts, A. W., Bokelman, D. L. *Fundam. Appl. Toxicol.* **16**, 320–329.

35 Sliskovic, D. R., Roth, B. D., Wilson, M. W., Hoefle, M. L., Newton, R. S. *J. Med. Chem.* **1990**, *33*, 31–38.

36 Sliskovic, D. R., Picard, J. A., Roark, Roth, B. D., W. H., Krause, B. R., Newton, R. S., Sekerke, C., Shaw, M. K. *J. Med. Chem.* **1991**, *34*, 367–373.

37 Reviewed in: Newton, D. M., Ramsden, C. A. *Tetrahedron* **1982**, *38*, 2965–3011.

38 Auerbach, B. J., Krause, B. R., Bisgaier, C. L., Newton, R. S. *Atherosclerosis (Shannon, Irel.)*, **1995**, *115*, 173–180.

39 Krause, B. R., Newton, R. S. *Atherosclerosis (Shannon, Irel.)* **1995**, *117*, 237–244.

40 Braun, M., Devant, R. *Tetrahedron Lett.* **1984**, 5031–5034.

41 Browner, P. L., Butler, D. E., Deering, C. F., Le, T. V., Millar, A., Nanninga, T. N., Roth, B. D. *Tetrahedron Lett.* **1992**, 2279–2282.

42 Baumann, K. L., Butler, D. E., Deering, C. F., Mennen, K. E., Millar, A., Nanninga, T. N., Palmer, C. W., Roth, B. D. *Tetrahedron Lett.* **1992**, 2283–2284.

43 Sletzinger, M., Verhoeven, T.R., McNamara, J. M., Corley, E. G., Lui, T. M. H. *Tetrahedron Lett.* **1985**, 2951–2955.

44 Isbell, H. S., Frush, H. L. *Carbohyd. Res.* **1979**, *72*, 301–304.

45 Bock, K., Lundt, I., Pedersen, C. *Acta Chem. Scand.* **1983**, *37B*, 341–344.

46 Brooks, D. W., Lu, L., D.-L., Masamune, S. *Angew. Chem. Int. Ed. Eng.* **1979**, *18*, 72.

47 Chen, K. M., Hardtmann, G. E., Prasad, K., Repic, O., Shapiro, M. J. *Tetrahedron Lett.* **1987**, 155–159.

48 Cilla, D. D., Posvar, E. L., Sedman, A. J. *J. Clin. Pharm.* **1992**, *32*, p. 749, abs. #28.

49 Nawrocki, J. W., Weiss, S. R., Davidson, M. H., Sprecher, D. L., Schwartz, S. L., Lupien, P.-J., Jones, P. H., Haber, H. H., Black, D. M. *Arterioscler. Thromb.* **1995**, *15*, 678–682.

50 Bakker-Arkema, R. G., Davidson, M. H., Goldstein, R. J., Davignon, J., Isaacson, J. L., Weiss, S. R., Keilson, L. M., Brown, W. V., Miller, V. T., Shurzinske, L. J., Black, D. M. *JAMA*, **1996**, *275*, 128–133.

51 Jones, P., Kafonek, S., Laurora, I., Hunninghake, D. for the CURVES Investigators. *Am. J. Cardiol.* **1998**, *81*, 582–587.

52 For a review see: Chong, P. H., Seeger, J. D. *Pharmacotherapy* **1997**, *17*, 1157–1177.

Progress in Medicinal Chemistry – Vol. 40,
Series Editors: F.D. King and A.W. Oxford
Guest Editors: A.B. Reitz and S.L. Dax

# 2 Discovery of CEP-1347/KT-7515, an Inhibitor of the JNK/SAPK Pathway for the Treatment of Neurodegenerative Diseases

MICHAEL S. SAPORITO, ROBERT L. HUDKINS[*1]
AND ANNA C. MARONEY

*Departments of Medicinal Chemistry[1] and Neurobiology
Cephalon Inc., 145 Brandywine Parkway
West Chester, PA 19380, U.S.A.*

## ABSTRACT

Apoptosis has been proposed as a mechanism of cell death in Alzheimer's, Huntington's and Parkinson's diseases and the occurrence of apoptosis in these disorders suggests a common mechanism. Events such as oxidative stress, calcium toxicity, mitochondria defects, excitatory toxicity, and deficiency of survival factors are all postulated to play varying roles in the pathogenesis of the diseases. However, the transcription factor c-jun may play a role in the pathology and cell death processes that occur in Alzheimer's disease. Parkinson's disease (PD) is also a progressive disorder involving the specific degeneration and death of dopamine neurons in the nigrostriatal pathway. In Parkinson's disease, dopaminergic neurons in the substantia nigra are hypothesized to undergo cell death by apoptotic processes. The commonality of biochemical events and pathways leading to cell death in these diseases continues to be an area under intense investigation. The current therapy for PD and AD remains targeting replacement of lost transmitter, but the ultimate objective in neurodegenerative therapy is the functional restoration and/or cessation of progression of neuronal loss. This chapter will describe a novel approach for the treatment of neurodegenerative diseases through the development of kinase inhibitors that block the active cell death process at an early transcriptional independent step in the stress activated kinase cascade. In particular, preclinical data will be presented on the c-Jun Amino Kinase pathway inhibitor, CEP-1347/KT-7515, with respect to it's properties that make it a desirable clinical candidate for treatment of various neurodegenerative diseases.

## 1 INTRODUCTION

Neuronal cell death occurs in multiple neurodegenerative diseases such as Alzheimer's, Parkinson's and Huntington diseases [1,2]. Until recently, little was known about the molecular mechanisms leading to neuronal cell loss. There is now accumulating evidence that neurons from diseased individuals undergo a molecular process termed programmed cell death (PCD) [3,4]. This process initially involves independent transcriptional events that vary and appear to be dependent upon both the stress stimuli and the cellular environment. Once these early signals are stimulated they converge at the level of transcriptional activation leading eventually to an elevation of pro-apoptotic Bcl2 family members, cytochrome C release from the mitochondria and cytokine-dependent caspase activation [5]. Ultimately, the morphological features of apoptosis may become evident, such as nuclear DNA degradation or fragmentation and cell membrane blebbing. Cell membrane integrity is maintained and dying cells are eliminated by phagocytosis in the absence of an inflammatory response. DNA damage and apoptosis can be detected in postmortem sections from Alzheimer's patients [6,7]. Conceptually, blocking the cell death process may have an impact on the clinical treatment of neurodegenerative diseases.

## 2  c-Jun N-TERMINAL KINASE PATHWAY IN NEURONAL CELL DEATH

The stress activated proteins kinases (SAPK), which include the p38 and c-Jun $NH_2$ Kinases (JNKs), belong to the Mitogen Activated Protein Kinase (MAPK) superfamily and respond to a variety of stimuli such as environmental stress, cytokines, or initiators of cell death [8]. Particularly, the JNK signaling cascade, leading to activation of the c-Jun transcription factor, has been implicated in certain neuronal pro-apoptotic responses dependent upon the cellular environment and stimulus.

The c-Jun transcription factor was first implicated in neuronal cell death by three independent approaches. Microinjection of neutralizing c-Jun antibody, antisense oligonucleotides or expression of a transactivation c-Jun mutant lacking the DNA binding domain prevents sympathetic and hippocampal neuronal cell death evoked by trophic factor deprivation or potassium depolarization [9–11]. Conversely, overexpression of c-Jun is sufficient to induce apoptosis of sympathetic neurons in the absence of an external insult [11].

The initial observations implicating c-Jun in neuronal cell death were followed by reports demonstrating that the kinases upstream of c-Jun activation can modulate the cell death response. The JNKs phosphorylate serine residues 63 and 73 of c-Jun, leading to its activation [12–14]. Preventing phosphorylation of these serine sites by mutating them to alanine protects differentiated PC12 cells and granule neurons from death due to trophic withdrawal or potassium depolarization, respectively [15,16]. The JNKs are activated by members of the MAPK kinase family, which include MKK4 and MKK7 [17–24]. Multiple kinase families upstream of the MKKs lead to JNK activation including the Mixed Lineage Kinase (MLK) and MEKK family, as well as Tpl-2, a member of the Raf family [25]. In particular, over expression of MEKK family members, such as MEKK1 or MEKK5/ASK1, induce death of differentiated PC12 cells [16,26,27]. Many of the MAPK kinase kinases contain a Cdc42/Rac interactive binding motif (CRIB) domain and regulation of these kinases is governed, in part, by binding to the small GTPases rac and cdc42 [28]. Constitutive activation of cdc42 can trigger death of sympathetic neurons [29].

Perhaps the most compelling data implicating the JNK/c-Jun pathway in neuronal apoptosis has emerged from gene targeting experiments. In JNK3 knockout mice, hippocampal neurons are protected from kainate induced cell death [30]. Notably, c-Jun dependent reporter activity is diminished in the JNK3 null background even though c-Jun gene induction continues to be elevated after kainate exposure, supporting the notion that the phosphorylation of c-Jun is critical in the regulation of its pro-apoptotic activity and not the level of c-Jun expression. Complementary to these results, hippocampal neurons from mice expressing c-jun with a serine to alanine mutation on sites 63 and 73 are also protected from kainate-induced cell death [31]. Taken together these data indicate that the JNK signaling cascade leading to phosphorylation of c-Jun is important in certain neuronal cell death processes.

Despite the *in vitro* and *in vivo* evidence described above, there is a great deal of debate on whether activation of c-Jun is pro-apoptotic or pro-survival in specific preclinical models of neurodegeneration. The literature presents persuasive evidence for each hypothesis. C-Jun expression is elevated by a variety of insults such as axotomy, excitotoxicity, hypoxia-ischemia and nerve crush [32–39]. The transient pattern of c-Jun expression parallels neuronal cell death in some instances, such as in transections of rat fimbria-fornix or ischemia. However, in others such as in axotomy or 6-hydroxydopamine lesions of the dopaminergic nigrostriatal pathway, it parallels regeneration [32,35,36,40,41]. Support for the dual function of c-Jun is further revealed from gene targeting experiments. Developmental programmed cell death occurs normally in c-Jun, phospho-c-Jun, JNK1, JNK2, and JNK3 null embryos [30,31,42–44]. However, a double deficiency of JNK1 and JNK2 results in embryonic lethality due to deregulated apoptosis during brain development [45]. These double knockout mice have regions of enhanced apoptosis such as in the hindbrain and regions of protection in the forebrain suggesting that JNK1 and JNK2 are involved in region-specific developmental programmed cell death in the brain [45].

Evidence implicating the JNK/c-Jun pathway in human neurodegenerative disease is limited. C-Jun immunoreactivity co-localizes with apoptotic bodies from tissue of Alzheimer's brains, and JNK phosphorylates Tau protein *in vitro* at sites that are hyperphosphorylated in Alzheimer's patients [46,47]. However, it remains to be determined whether inhibiting the JNK/c-Jun pathway will prevent human neuronal cell loss.

## 3 SURVIVAL PROMOTING PROPERTIES OF K-252a

K-252a (**1**, *Figure 2.1*), an indolocarbazole alkaloid isolated from *Nocardiopsis sp.*, [48] is an inhibitor of a number of serine/threonine and protein tyrosine kinases [49]. K-252a has also been reported to demonstrate "neurotrophic-like" or survival promoting properties [50]. For example, K-252a promotes neurite outgrowth in human SH-SY5Y neuroblastoma cells [51]. In primary cultures of embryonic neurons, K-252a promoted survival of dorsal root and ciliary ganglion neurons [52], enhanced ChAT (choline acetyltransferase) activity in spinal cord [53] and basal forebrain cultures [54] and promoted survival and ChAT activity in striatal cultures [55]. The neurotrophic activity demonstrated by K-252a for enhancing ChAT activity in spinal cord cultures was comparable to responses elicited by neurotrophic factors such as CNTF, BDNF and IGF-I (see *Figure 2.3*). Studies have shown K-252a protects neurons against glucose deprivation [55], free-radical induced injury and amyloid $\beta$-peptide toxicity [56].

The aglycone K-252c **2** (*Figure 2.1*) and further simplified carbazoles **3** and **4** were evaluated for their ability to promote ChAT activity in spinal cord cultures [57]. The aglycone **2** retained approximately 10–15% of K-252a activity while carbazole **3** was 10-fold weaker and **4** was inactive.

In contrast to its survival promoting properties, K-252a also inhibits NGF-induced neuronal differentiation and survival [58,59] by inhibiting NGFs high affinity receptor tyrosine kinase, trk A, as well as trks B and C [60–64]. In addition to inhibition of trk A tyrosine kinase with an $IC_{50} = 2.4$ nM, [65,66] K-

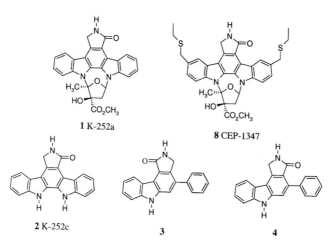

*Figure 2.1. The structures of indolocarbazoles.*

252a potently inhibits protein kinase C (PKC, $IC_{50} = 28\,nM$), cyclic AMP dependent protein kinase (PKA, $IC_{50} = 16\,nM$) and myosin light chain kinase (MLCK, $IC_{50} = 20\,nM$) [65,67].

## 4 K-252a ANALOGS

The biological profile of K-252a suggested that the development of compounds from the K-252a class as "survival promoting" agents may lead to an effective therapy for the treatment of certain peripheral and central neurodegenerative diseases. Medicinal chemistry efforts focused on a series of K-252a analogs, with the goal of selectively enhancing the ChAT activity in spinal cord and basal forebrain culture from the NGF (trk A tyrosine kinase) and protein kinase C inhibitory activities [65]. Analogs were screened for their ability to promote ChAT activity in embryonic rodent spinal cord [53] and basal forebrain [54] cultures. In the spinal cord, motor neurons are cholinergic and express ChAT. ChAT activity has been used in great detail to study the effects of neurotrophins (e.g., NGF or NT-3) on the survival and/or function of cholinergic neurons. Similar to the response of basal forebrain neurons to NGF, spinal cord motor neurons also respond to several other growth factors by increasing ChAT activity (*Figure 2.3*). In spinal cord cultures (E14-E19), a significant number of cholinergic neurons would be expected to die in the absence of a motoneuron survival factor. A continual decline in ChAT activity is observed with increasing culture time. In addition to spinal cord, basal forebrain neurons have also been identified as a K-252a-responsive neuronal population, showing increasing survival and ChAT activity. The history of K-252a in these assays rendered it a reliable and effective reference standard. In the spinal cord ChAT assay, K-252a shows a maximum enhancement of ChAT activity of $186 \pm 3\%$ above basal levels (100%) at 300 nM and is ineffective at concentrations below 100 nM. In the basal forebrain assay, K-252a is effective at concentrations as low as 50 nM (175% enhancement of ChAT), and shows a maximum effect of $325 \pm 22\%$ at 200 nM.

A set of 3,9-bis[(alkoxy)methyl] and 3,9-bis[(alkylthio)methyl] analogs were reported with potent and selective survival-promoting properties [65]. The data presented in *Table 2.1* show the 3,9-bis[(alkylthio)methyl] and 3,9-bis[(alkoxy)methyl] analogs were active in both the basal forebrain and spinal cord ChAT assays. The ethylthiomethyl derivative **8** (CEP-1347) displayed efficacy and potency at low concentrations in both spinal cord and basal forebrain ChAT assays. Substitutions demonstrate that alkyl groups larger than ethyl (CEP-1347 **8**) resulted in a decrease in potency (see **10–13**) in these assays. Bis[(alkylthio)methyl] substitution enhanced efficacy (over K-252a) in the spinal cord

Table 2.1. ACTIVITY OF 3,9-DISUBSTITUTED K-252a DERIVATIVES

| Compound | R | Spinal Cord ChAT % of control[a] | | Basal Forebrain ChAT % of control[a] | | trk A IC$_{50}$ (nM)[c] |
|---|---|---|---|---|---|---|
| | | 30 nM | 300 nM | 50 nM | 250 nM | |
| 1 (K-252a) | H | < 120 | 186 ± 3 | 148 ± 10 | 325 ± 22[d] | 2.4 |
| 5 | CH$_2$OH | < 120 | < 120 | nt[b] | nt[b] | nt[b] |
| 6 | CH$_2$OMe | 193 ± 11 | 218 ± 14 | 168 ± 12 | 340 ± 21 | 270 |
| 7 | CH$_2$OEt | 153 ± 17 | 188 ± 20 | < 120 | 237 ± 22 | 210 |
| 8 | CH$_2$SEt | 140 ± 8 | 280 ± 14 | 143 ± 15 | 363 ± 26 | >1000 |
| 9 | CH$_2$S$^n$Pr | < 120 | 315 ± 20 | < 120 | 180 ± 6 | >1000 |
| 10 | CH$_2$S$^i$Pr | < 120 | 289 ± 17 | nt[b] | 224 ± 24 | >1000 |
| 11 | CH$_2$SCH$_2$CH=CH$_2$ | < 120 | 302 ± 12 | < 120 | 191 ± 12 | >1000 |
| 12 | CH$_2$S$^n$Bu | < 120 | 289 ± 6 | 143 ± 8 | 200 ± 19 | >1000 |
| 13 | CH$_2$SCH$_2$CH$_2$NMe$_2$ | < 120 | 208 ± 8 | < 120 | 158 ± 15 | nt[b] |

[a]Enhancement of ChAT activity versus untreated control cultures.
[b]nt = not tested.
[c]Concentration required to inhibit 50% of *trk* kinase.
[d]>200 nM conc. decreases ChAT below basal levels.

ChAT assay while in basal forebrain cultures, except for CEP-1347 **8**, reduced efficacy was observed.

The dose response for K-252a and CEP-1347 for enhancing ChAT in spinal cord cultures is shown in *Figure 2.2*. K-252a displays a decrease in ChAT activity above 200 nM in culture, as opposed to CEP-1347, which did not display this inverted dose response curve at micromolar concentrations (*Figure 2.2*) [65].

An important discovery to achieve kinase selectivity was that the bis-ether derivatives **6** (IC$_{50}$ = 270 nM) and **7** (IC$_{50}$ = 210 nM) were about 100-fold weaker than K-252a in inhibition for trk A tyrosine kinase, while the alkylthiomethyl analogs (**10–13**) displayed IC$_{50}$ values>1 µM (*Table 2.1*). This information suggested that proper substitution in the 3- and 9-positions reduces or eliminates trk A kinase inhibitory activity >500-fold while enhancing the neuronal "survival-promoting" properties in culture. This was a critical discovery for development of a small molecule survival agent. As shown in *Table 2.2*, in comparison to K-252a, CEP-1347 did not inhibit protein kinase C

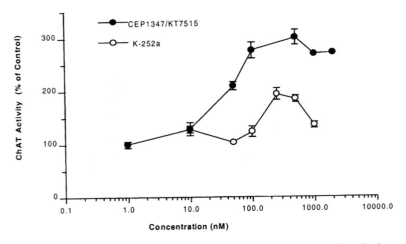

*Figure 2.2.   Enhancement of ChAT activity by CEP-1347 and K-252a in spinal cord cultures.*

Table 2.2.   INHIBITORY EFFECT OF CEP-1347 ON VARIOUS KINASES

|  | $IC_{50}(\mu M)$ | |
| --- | --- | --- |
| Kinase | *K-252a* | *Compound CEP 1347* |
| Protein kinase C[a] | 0.028 | 16.3 |
| cAMP-dependent protein kinase[b] | 0.016 | >10 |
| Myosin light chain kinase[c] | 0.02 | >10 |

[a]C-kinase was prepared from rat brain.
[b]A-kinase was prepared from rabbit skeletal muscle.
[c]MLCK was prepared from chicken gizzard.

(PKC), cAMP-dependant protein kinase (PKA) and myosin light chain kinase (MLCK) with $IC_{50}$ values $>10\,\mu M$ [65].

## 5  DISCOVERY OF CEP-1347

### 5.1  *IN VITRO* ACTIVITY IN PERIPHERAL AND CENTRAL NEURONS

CEP-1347 was more potent and efficacious than K-252a for enhancement of ChAT activity in spinal cord cultures [65] (*Figure 2.2*). Under the experimental conditions used, CEP-1347 is equal to or more efficacious in promoting spinal

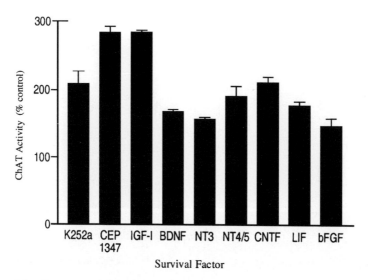

*Figure 2.3.* Comparison of CEP-1347 **8** and K-252a **1** with various survival factors on the enhancement of ChAT activity in spinal cord culture.

cord ChAT activity when compared to neurotrophic protein growth factors (*Figure 2.3*).

The increase in ChAT activity by CEP-1347 in spinal cord cultures was associated with promotion of long-term survival of neurons derived from embryonic chick dorsal root sympathetic and ciliary ganglia, and embryonic chick and rodent motor neurons [68,69]. At maximum effective concentrations, CEP-1347 (300 nM) enhanced chick motor neuron survival over untreated controls by 79%, compared to 28% survival by K-252a (150 nM) [68]. In addition to promotion of survival of embryonic neurons from the peripheral and central nervous system, CEP-1347 also produced robust neurite outgrowth [68].

### 5.2 MECHANISM OF ACTION

To elucidate the mechanism by which CEP-1347 promoted survival of embryonic neurons *in vitro*, purified motor neurons from rat spinal cord tissue were examined in the presence of CEP-1347 after trophic withdrawal. Lack of trophic support induces apoptosis in motor neurons [70,71]. Treatment of trophic deprived motor neurons with CEP-1347 blocked the appearance of condensed nuclei and prevented neurite retraction (*Figure 2.4*). CEP-1347 promoted motor neuronal survival comparable to that elicited by optimal concentrations of protein growth factors [72–76].

CONTROL                              250 nM CEP1347

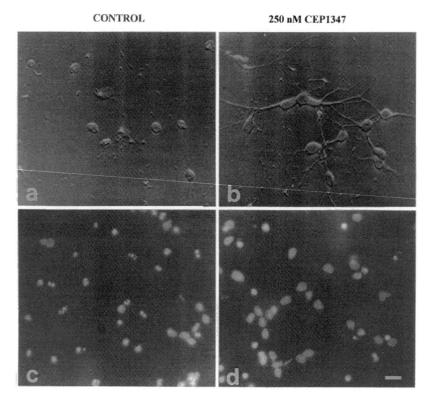

*Figure 2.4.   Apoptosis of enriched E14.5 motor neurons in the absence or presence of CEP-1347.*
*Cells were plated at a density of $6 \times 10^4$ cells/cm² in chemically defined N2 medium. After 2 hr to*
*allow for attachment control cells were incubated with 0.006% DMSO control (a, c) or 250 nM*
*CEP-1347 (b, d) for 5d followed by fixation and photography using Hoffman modulating contrast*
*optics (a, b) or for 2d followed by staining with Hoechst dye (c, d) to detect condensed chromatin.*
*Copyright 1999 by the Society for Neuroscience.*

In order to initially determine the molecular mechanism by which CEP-1347 elicited neuronal survival, the MAPK signaling cascade was examined since many survival and death stimuli converge at this level of signal transduction. Of the three MAPK families (ERK, p38 and JNK), the cascade leading to ERK activation has been implicated in neuronal survival [26]. The basal level of ERK1 activity did not change in motor neurons after trophic withdrawal, and therefore CEP-1347 promoted survival in the absence of a change in ERK1 activity [76]. Furthermore, CEP-1347 did not suppress ERK activation induced by treatment of motoneurons with brain-derived growth factor (unpublished results). In contrast, JNK1 activity increased approximately 4-fold within 24 hr after trophic withdrawal. CEP-1347 markedly decreased the JNK1 activity in a dose dependent manner (*Figure 2.5*). Irradiation, sorbitol and tunicamycin can induce JNK activity [13,14,77,78]. The effect on inhibition of JNK1 activation was an intrinsic property of CEP-1347 since CEP-1347 significantly attenuated JNK1 activation by these insults in Cos-7 cells (*Table 2.3*). Therefore, inhibition of JNK1 activation by CEP-1347 was not neuronal or stimuli specific. The concentration of CEP-1347 to inhibit 50% of JNK1 activity ($IC_{50}$) was comparable to the concentration to produce a half maximal response for survival ($EC_{50}$ 20 nM) by CEP-1347, suggesting that these two activities were related.

Activation of p38, another MAPK family in the stress pathway, has also been implicated in neuronal cell death [26]. To determine whether CEP-1347 could affect p38, the activity of a substrate of p38, MAPKAP2, was examined in Cos-7 cells subjected to osmotic shock, a treatment that has been previously shown to activate p38 [79,80]. CEP-1347 did not affect MAPKAP2 activity (*Table 2.3*, 76). In contrast, the p38 inhibitor SB203580 completely blocked the osmotic stress-induced p38 activity [81,76]. These results demonstrated that CEP-1347 did not effect p38 directly or upstream regulators of the osmotic shock-induced MAPKAP2 activity.

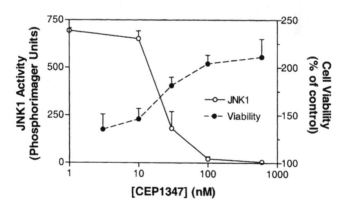

*Figure 2.5. Dose response of inhibition of JNK1 activity and cell survival by CEP-1347. Cultures of enriched E14.5 motor neurons were plated and allowed to adhere 2.5 hr prior to addition of the indicated concentrations of CEP-1347. For JNK1 activity, cells were collected 22 hr after addition of compound and assayed for kinase activity with c-Jun substrate;cell viability was determined by Calcein-AM assay after 5 days in culture. Percent of cell viability is relative to untreated controls, which is equivalent to 100%. Points represent the average of duplicate samples where the error bar indicates the standard error of the mean. Copyright 1999 by the Society for Neuroscience.*

Table 2.3.   Activity of CEP-1347 Subjected to Osmotic Shock
A. JNK1 Activity in Stressed-Induced Cos7 cells[a]

| Treatment | Control | CEP-1347 |
|---|---|---|
| Untreated | 1.0 | 1.0 |
| Irradiation | 5.3 | 2.4 |
| Sorbitol | 7.8 | 2.4 |
| Tunicamycin | 1.6 | 0.9 |

B. MAPKAP2 Activity in Osmotic Shocked Cos7 cells

| Treatment | Control | CEP-1347 | SB203580 |
|---|---|---|---|
| Untreated | 1.0 | 1.4 | 0.6 |
| Sorbitol | 8.1 | 7.6 | 1.0 |

[a]Cells were grown to confluency and pretreated with DMSO, 500 nM CEP-1347 or 10 $\mu$M SB203580 for 1 hr prior to treatment with U.V. irradiation (5 min in Stratolinker followed by 1 hr incubation at 37°C), sorbitol (500 mM sorbitol for 1 hr) or tunicamycin (50 ug/ml for 5 hr). Lysates were collected, normalized for protein and immunoprecipitated with the JNK1 (A) or MAPKAP2 (B) antibody and assayed for kinase activity. Results are expressed as the fold increase relative to untreated control. Copyright 1998 by the Society for Neuroscience.

Loss of trophic support, DNA damage and oxidative stress are among the insults that may lead to neuronal cell death in disease [82–84]. CEP-1347 was evaluated under these various stresses to determine its effect on neuronal survival as well as JNK activation in sympathetic neurons cultured from newborn rats and PC12 cells. CEP-1347 prevented the death of both cell populations after NGF withdrawal, UV irradiation or treatment with antisense to superoxide dismutase-1 in a dose dependent manner (*Figure 2.6A*) [85]. Maximum rescue was observed at 100 nM CEP-1347 similar to survival activity in motor neurons [85].

Given the observation that CEP-1347 blocked JNK activation in motor neurons, it was of interest to determine whether the mechanism of action of CEP-1347 also correlated with inhibition of JNK activation after loss of trophic support, DNA damage or oxidative stress in differentiated PC12 cells. As demonstrated previously in multiple models [26,86,13,87,88], these insults led to activation of JNK within 4–6 hrs of treatment [85]. In each insult, the increase in JNK activation was blocked by CEP-1347 (*Figure 2.6B*). Comparable results were obtained whether total JNK activity was measured or phosphorylation of the p46 and p54 JNK isoforms. In both measurements, the level of total JNK activity/phosphorylation was below basal levels after treatment with CEP-1347 at concentrations greater than 30 nM. Thus, as in motor neuron cultures, the

**A.**

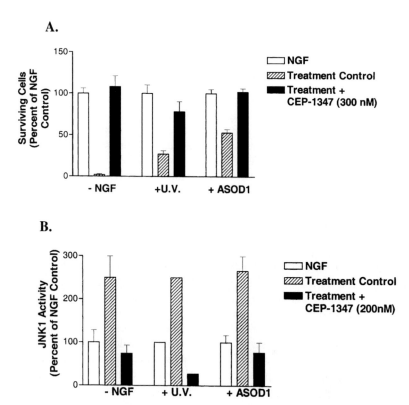

**B.**

*Figure 2.6. Effect of CEP-1347 on the survival and JNK activation of differentiated PC12 cells after distinct insults. (A) Differentiated PC12 cells maintained in NGF were assessed for cell survival four days after withdrawal of NGF or two days after UV irradiation or treatment with antisense to superoxide dismutase-1 in the absence (lanes 1 and 2) or presence of 300 nM CEP-1347 (lane 3). The percentage of cell survival is expressed relative to NGF-treated controls (lane 1). Data shown are the mean ± SEM of triplicate wells. (B) JNK1 activity was measured at times of peak activation four hours after withdrawal of NGF or six hours after UV irradiation or treatment with antisense to superoxide dismutase-1 in the absence (lanes 1 and 2) or presence of 200 nM CEP-1347 (lane 3). Cell lysates were collected, normalized to protein, immunoprecipitated with a JNK1 antibody and assayed for JNK1 activity. The level of JNK1 activity is expressed relative to the time-matched NGF-treated control (given as 100%). Each bar represents the average of duplicate samples; error bars indicate range. Reproduced from Journal of Neurochemistry, 1999, with permission.*

mechanism of action of CEP-1347's survival promoting activity appeared to be associated with inhibition of JNK activation.

Previous reports have demonstrated that death evoked by trophic withdrawal, DNA damage and oxidative stress involve distinct downstream targets [86,89–

91]. For example, cyclin-dependent kinase inhibitors can protect from death caused by NGF deprivation and DNA damage but not oxidative stress. Moreover, cyclic AMP protects from death due to trophic factor deprivation, but has no effect in SOD1 depletion or DNA damage. Inhibitors of caspase 1 (ICE, interleukin-1β converting enzyme) prevent death due to SOD1 depletion, whereas, down-regulation of caspase 2 (Nedd2) suppresses death evoked by NGF withdrawal. Notwithstanding these divergences in overall mechanism, there appears to be a shared component to all three death pathways that is blocked by CEP-1347 and these results suggest that the shared component is activation of the JNK pathway.

The association between CEP-1347's inhibitory activity against JNK activation and promotion of survival is not universal. CEP-1347 did not rescue naïve PC12 cells at concentrations that inhibited JNK activation [85]. Furthermore, Fas activation of Jurkat human T-cells via the CD40 receptor leads to activation of JNK and subsequent cell death [92]. However, the role of JNK in mediating this death is controversial [88,93–98]. Jurkat cells treated with anti-Fas antibody to activate the CD40 receptor in the presence of CEP-1347 were not rescued at concentrations up 3 μM even though JNK activation was completely blocked by 200 nM CEP-1347 [85]. Hence, as with naive PC12 cells, CEP-1347 has poor survival-promoting activity on Fas-treated Jurkat cells, but effectively blocks activation of JNK1. These data support that JNK activation is neither sufficient nor necessary for all apoptotic cell death. Overall, the molecular mechanism by which CEP-1347 elicits neuronal survival is consistent with inhibition of the JNK pathway [76]. Although the target(s) of CEP-1347 in the JNK pathway are still under investigation, results indicate CEP-1347 potently inhibits the mixed lineage kinase family members while it does not inhibit MEKK1 activated JNK1. GST-tagged truncated kinase-active forms of three MLK members (MLK1, MLK2, MLK3) were expressed and purified from insect cells infected with baculovirus constructs expressing these proteins. Kinase assays were established using myelin basic protein as a substrate. CEP-1347 displayed potently inhibition *in vitro* with $IC_{50}$ values of 38, 51, and 23 nM for MLK1, MLK2, and MLK3, respectively (Maroney, A.C et al. *J. Biol. Chem.* submitted). These inhibitory values were in the same range of the $IC_{50}$ values obtained using cells co-expressing full-length MLK family members and a substrate, dnMKK4. The mode of inhibition of MLK1 with respect to ATP was consistent with competitive type kinetics for CEP-1347 versus ATP.

## 5.3 *IN VIVO* ACTIVITY IN MOTORNEURON MODELS

The enhancement of ChAT activity and motor neuronal survival in spinal cord cultures suggests potential utility in various motor neuron diseases such as amyotrophic lateral sclerosis (ALS) and certain peripheral neuropathies.

A broad assessment of motor neuronal survival properties of CEP-1347 was made in which the age of the animal, motor neuron location and mode of death were distinct [99]. Approximately 50% of vertebrate motor neurons undergo programmed cell death during embryogenesis. It is hypothesized that this is due in part to a limited supply of target derived survival factors. In the chick, 40–50% of the lumbar motor neurons die between embryonic days E6 and E10 [100]. To examine potential effects on neuronal programmed cell death, doses of CEP-1347 were delivered locally onto the chorioallantoic membrane surrounding the embryo from E6-E9, followed by embryo sacrifice on E10. Maximally effective doses of 2.3 and 7 µg/day/egg of CEP-1347 rescued 40% (of the 50%) of the motor neurons that would normally die during this period.

In a second model, CEP-1347 was effective at rescuing motor neurons of the spinal nucleus of the bulbocavernosus (SNB). In female rats, SNB neurons die postnatally due to the absence of steroid hormone, a required non-protein survival factor [101]. From birth to postnatal day (PN) 4 in the female rat approximately 50% of the motor neurons of the sexually dimorphic SNB are eliminated by programmed cell death. CEP-1347 (1 mg/kg/sc) attenuated motor neuron death with efficacy equal to that in testosterone controls [101].

Axonal injury often results in morphological as well as biochemical changes in the injured nerve cell body [102]. CEP-1347 was assessed in a third model of motor neuronal degeneration, axotomy of the hypoglossal nerve in the adult rat. CEP-1347 dose-dependently attenuated the decrease in hypoglossal motor neuron-ChAT immunoreactivity assessed 7 days post axotomy compared to the axotomized, untreated control.

## 5.4 *IN VIVO* ACTIVITY IN ANIMAL MODELS OF CHOLINERGIC DEGENERATION

A basis for selecting *in vivo* animal models for evaluation of CEP-1347 was efficacy of a specific cell type in cell culture. One cell type that was affected by CEP-1347 was cholinergic neurons derived from embryonic basal forebrain [65]. Magnocellular cholinergic neurons that originate in the basal forebrain and project to the cortex and the hippocampus are implicated in cognitive function in rodents and in primates, including humans [103–106]. In Alzheimer's disease (AD), there is marked degeneration of the cortically projecting cholinergic neurons of the nucleus basalis of Meynert (NBM) that may be associated with certain cognitive deficits of the disease [107]. Theoretically, a drug that prevented the degeneration of basal forebrain cholinergic neurons could slow or halt development of cognitive deficits in AD patients.

A variety of adult animal models have been established that attempt to replicate the cholinergic neuronal deficits that occur in AD [108,109]. These models do not attempt to simulate the neuropathology of AD, but simply attempt to replicate the cholinergic loss that is seen in the disease [110]. Animal models of cholinergic degeneration have proven vital in assessing the cognitive enhancing ability of agents that increase cholinergic transmission, restore cholinergic function or prevent cholinergic neuronal degeneration [106,111,112].

### 5.4.1 Activity of CEP-1347 in the NBM Lesion Model

The NBM lesion model involves excitotoxic injury of cortically projecting cholinergic neurons that lie within the region that correspond to the cortically projecting cholinergic neurons of the nucleus basalis of Meynert in humans. In human AD these neurons degenerate and their loss is thought to contribute to some of the cognitive deficits seen in the disease [103,107,113,114]. Administration of an NMDA agonist (ibotenic acid) directly to the NBM produces a loss of cortically projecting cholinergic nerve terminals as measured by a loss of choline acetyltransferase activity (ChAT), loss of ChAT immunoreactivity and cell death [115–117].

The neuronal survival properties of CEP-1347 were characterized in the NBM lesion model [116]. Peripheral administration of CEP-1347 at subcutaneous doses between 0.1 and 1.0 mg/kg attenuated the ibotenic acid-mediated degeneration of cortically-projecting cholinergic neurons as measured

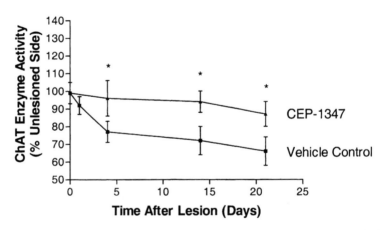

Figure 2.7. Time course of the effects of CEP-1347 in the NBM lesion model. CEP-1347 (0.1 mg/kg/dose) was administered 6 hr prior to the lesion, 18 hrs post-lesion and then every 48 hrs until the indicated time. ChAT activity in the frontal cortex was assessed at the indicated times after lesion. Values are expressed as the averages ± SEM, of the ratio of ChAT activity on the lesioned side to that on the unlesioned side (Ipsilateral/Contralateral Ratio × 100). *Indicates statistical difference (p < 0.05) from vehicle treated control at the same time point.

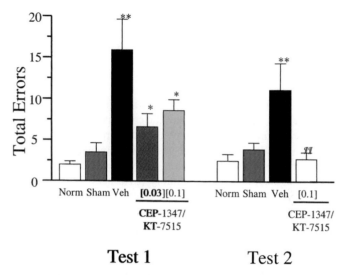

Test 1                    Test 2

*Figure 2.8. CEP-1347 attenuates cognitive impairment associated with lesioning of the nucleus basalis mgnocellularis. Total incorrect arm alternations (errors) during each of two post-operative tests: Test 1, beginning 13 days post-lesioning of the NBM and Test 2, beginning 8–10 weeks after completion of Test 1 (10–12 weeks post-dosing). Both tests consisted of 8 trials/day and continued until pre-operative performance level was reached. CEP-1347 animals received either 0.03 or 0.1 mg/kg of the drug q.o.d. over the first 12 post-operative days. Values are means ± s.e.m. ** P < 0.01 vs. SHAM, * P < 0.05 vs. VEH,¶¶ P < 0.01 vs. VEH, Newman-Keuls tests following separate ANOVA for each test.*

by cortical ChAT enzyme activity and ChAT immunoreactivity in the NBM. The neuronal survival properties of CEP-1347 in the NBM lesion model were distinct from the neurotrophic characteristics of NGF. For instance, CEP-1347 attenuated the loss of frontal cortex ChAT activity as soon as the loss was fully detectable, whereas centrally administered NGF only increased cortical ChAT activity with 14 days of continuous infusion. Furthermore, CEP-1347 did not restore ChAT activity with delayed administration indicating that, unlike NGF, CEP-1347 did not increase the expression of cholinergic functional parameters. The data were interpreted to indicate that the biochemical efficacy of CEP-1347 in this model was principally due to prevention of excitotoxin-induced neurodegeneration of cortically projecting cholinergic neurons [116].

In addition to preventing the loss of the biochemical marker, ChAT, CEP-1347 administration attenuated the ibotenic acid-mediated loss of cholinergic cell bodies, as measured by ChAT immunoreactive cell number in the NBM [116]. The CEP-1347 mediated preservation corresponded with preservation of NBM neurons retrogradely labeled with fluorogold [117], indicating that

CEP-1347 prevented the injury-induced loss of the phenotypic marker ChAT and prevented injury-induced cell death.

### 5.4.2 Effects of CEP-1347 on Cognitive Function in the NBM Lesion Model

Direct lesioning of the NBM in rodents and in primates produces behavioral and cognitive deficits that reflect some of the cognitive dysfunction seen in AD. More refined behavioral analyses coupled with more selective lesioning techniques in animal models of AD have led to the conclusion that the primary functional role of the NBM, at least in monkeys and rodents, involves aspects of attention rather than short-term memory [118–122]. More recently, neurological studies have highlighted a loss in directed (cognitive) attention as an early symptom of AD [123,124]. Direct infusion of protein growth factors such as NGF into the CNS increases cholinergic functional markers and improves learning and memory functions in animals with injured cholinergic neurons of the NBM [112,125–128].

In order to test whether the cholinergic neurons in this NBM lesion model were maintained in a functional state with CEP-1347 treatment, CEP-1347 was assessed for the ability to attenuate cognitive deficits evoked by destruction of NBM cholinergic neurons [129]. The task used for testing rats with NBM lesions was a delayed alternation in a T-maze task, which is a spatial version of the delayed-nonmatch-to-position type of task used to assess short-term memory in monkeys and rodents [130]. Subcutaneous administration of CEP-1347 improved accuracy in a delayed nonmatch-to-position test in adult rats with ibotenic acid lesions of the NBM [129]. The improvement was seen after twelve days of dosing, and then again in the same animals 10–12 weeks after dosing had ceased, at which point there was no difference in performance between the treated animals and controls. The behavioral results demonstrated that the magnitude and nature of the neuroprotection at the level of biochemical and morphological markers was sufficient to attenuate the lesion-induced cognitive impairment associated with loss of NBM cholinergic neurons and that the preserved cholinergic neurons remained functional.

### 5.4.3 Activity of CEP-1347 in the Fimbria-Fornix Model

The fimbria-fornix rodent model of basal forebrain cholinergic deficiency involves the direct mechanical transection of the septo-hippocampal pathway [130–132] and differs from the NBM model in that transection of the afferent cholinergic pathway results in a retrograde degeneration of basal forebrain cholinergic neurons in the septum and loss of hippocampal cholinergic terminals [131–133]. The advantage and utility of this lesion model is that these

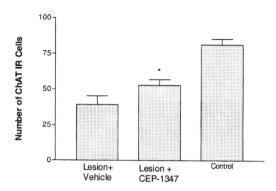

*Figure 2.9. Quantification of the number of cholinergic neurons in the medial septum following fimbria-fornix transection. CEP-1347 was continuously infused via subcutaneously implanted osmotic minipump at a dose of 0.25 mg/kg/day. ChAT immunoreactive neurons were counted throughout the medial septum. \* Indicates statistically significant difference from control.*

cholinergic neurons are morphologically similar to the magnocellular cholinergic neurons of the NBM and are anatomically organized in a well-defined fashion within the septum [105]. Moreover, the afferent projection pathway is tightly contained within the fimbria-fornix, which permits relatively easy surgical transection [105,134]. Finally, the fimbria-fornix transection model is well characterized for its responsiveness to the trophic activity of NGF and other trophic factors [131,132,135,136].

CEP-1347 administration attenuated the loss of septo-hippocampal cholinergic neurons following transection of the fimbria-fornix [133]. The protection occurred by either subcutaneous daily administration of CEP-1347 (1 mg/kg/dose) or by infusion with a subcutaneous implanted osmotic minipump (0.25 mg/kg/day). The extent of neuroprotection seen with CEP-1347 was similar to the effects observed with brain derived neurotrophic factor (BDNF) and glial derived neurotrophic factor (GDNF) in a similar model of septo-hippocampal transection [135,136]. However, the neuroprotective efficacy was lower than the neuroprotection detected on treatment with NGF, which protects approximately 80–90% of cholinergic neurons in the medial septum [136,137]. Studies of CEP-1347 in the fimbria-fornix lesion model indicated that the neuroprotective activity on cholinergic neurons was not isolated to models utilizing excitotoxic injury.

5.5 PARKINSON'S DISEASE AND MPTP MODELS OF NEURODEGENERATION

Parkinson's disease is a neurodegenerative disease that displays well-characterized neuropathological, behavioral and mechanistic characteristics.

In Parkinson's disease there is a well-defined, slowly progressing, relatively selective loss of nigrostriatal dopaminergic neurons [138,139]. The loss of dopaminergic neurons is the primary cause of the hallmark locomotor deficits (bradykinesia, tremor, postural instability) associated with this disease [138–140]. Moreover, reversal of these locomotor deficits can be elicited by administration of dopamimetic drugs and agents that increase CNS levels of dopamine [141,142]. The characteristic features of the disease suggest that a drug capable of attenuating nigrostriatal dopaminergic degeneration and subsequently maintained dopaminergic tone would theoretically slow or halt the progressive nature of the disease.

The animal models of PD are more advanced and better characterized than animal models for other neurodegenerative diseases. The best characterized and most relevant animal models of PD utilize the selective nigrostriatal dopaminergic neurotoxin 1-methyl-4-phenyl-tetrahydropyridine (MPTP). MPTP administration to experimental animals produces a remarkable neuropathology similarity to idiopathic human PD [139,143–146]. These similarities allow the rational study of neurodegenerative mechanisms and permit the extension of findings to neurodegenerative mechanisms in human PD.

Understanding the mechanism of MPTP neurotoxicity is critical in interpreting the results of neuroprotective compounds in MPTP animal models. The dopaminergic neurotoxicity of MPTP is well-characterized and is dependent on the monoamine oxidase B (MAO-B)-mediated 2-electron oxidation of MPTP to $MPP^+$ in the CNS [143], active uptake of $MPP^+$ into dopaminergic neurons via the dopamine transporter [147–149], accumulation of $MPP^+$ in mitochondria, [148] and inhibition of complex I of the electron transport chain [149–151]. Drugs that inhibit MAO-B or dopamine uptake produce neuroprotective activity in MPTP-models of degeneration [143,147]. The key mechanistic similarities between MPTP-mediated neurotoxicity and idiopathic PD revolve around the mitochondrial deficiencies seen in both the disease and MPTP-intoxicated animals. $MPP^+$ ultimately damages dopaminergic neurons by inhibiting complex I of the mitochondrial electron transport chain [148–150,152]. In idiopathic PD, complex I deficiencies have been identified in the substantia nigra of PD patients and these deficiencies may be sufficient to precipitate neurodegeneration in the disease [153,154]. The similarities between MPTP-induced neurotoxicity and idiopathic PD indicate that MPTP produces a mechanistically relevant model of PD. Thus, events secondary to $MPP^+$ inhibition of mitochondrial respiration may be applicable to neurodegenerative events that occur in PD.

Programmed cell death mechanisms, secondary to complex I deficiencies, may play a role in the neurodegenerative processes in MPTP-induced toxicity and PD. In cell culture systems MPTP ($MPP^+$) produces morphological features of apoptosis including nuclear chromatin condensation and membrane blebbing, as well as DNA laddering in PC12 cells, SH-SY5Y cells, cultured mesencephalic neurons and cerebellar granule cells. Moreover, administration of MPTP to mice produces morphological characteristics of apoptosis in the substantia nigra [155–159]. Several intraneuronal pathways of programmed cell death have been implicated in MPTP-induced neurotoxicity. Mice over-expressing $BCL_2$ (an anti-apoptotic protein) or deficient in p53 (a pro-apoptotic protein) are resistant to MPTP-induced neurotoxicity [160,161]. Interestingly, nuclear chromatin condensation, and an increase in the nuclear translocation of NF-kappa B were found in the substantia nigra from PD patients, suggesting that programmed cell death mechanisms may participate in dopaminergic neurodegeneration in the disease [162,163]. These findings clearly described the potential association of programmed cell death pathways in dopaminergic neurodegeneration in both MPTP-intoxicated animals and suggested (along with the morphological evidence) that these apoptotic events could be occurring in PD. The identification of various apoptotic mechanisms occurring in MPTP-induced dopaminergic degeneration suggested the possibility that the apoptotic JNK signaling cascade may also be activated and associated with this neuronal injury event.

Based on these observations, the neuroprotective activity of CEP-1347 in MPTP-treated mice and subsequently non-human primates was investigated. Studies were also conducted to investigate this possibility and characterize the activation of the JNK signaling pathway in the nigrostriatal system in mice.

### 5.5.1 Neuroprotective Activity of CEP-1347 in MPTP-Treated Mice

The MPTP mouse model is a well-described animal model of PD. Systemic administration of MPTP to mice destroys dopaminergic terminals and, under appropriate dosing and timing conditions, destroys dopaminergic cell bodies in the substantia nigra. Under MPTP dosing conditions in which MPTP selectively destroyed striatal dopaminergic terminals without affecting dopaminergic cell bodies, systemic administration of CEP-1347 significantly attenuated the MPTP-mediated decrease in all striatal dopaminergic terminal parameters [164]. Under conditions in which MPTP damaged dopaminergic cell bodies in the substantia nigra, CEP-1347 administration attenuated the loss of these MPTP-damaged neurons (*Figure 2.10*).

These data indicated that CEP-1347 protected both degenerating dopaminergic cell bodies and striatal nerve terminals. The effective dose range of 0.03–3 mg/kg/dose was similar for the striatal and substantia nigra measures, suggesting that the neuroprotective activities of CEP-1347 on both dopaminergic parameters were related. Moreover, the CEP-1347 dose range for neuroprotection in the MPTP model was similar to the range for neuroprotection in the

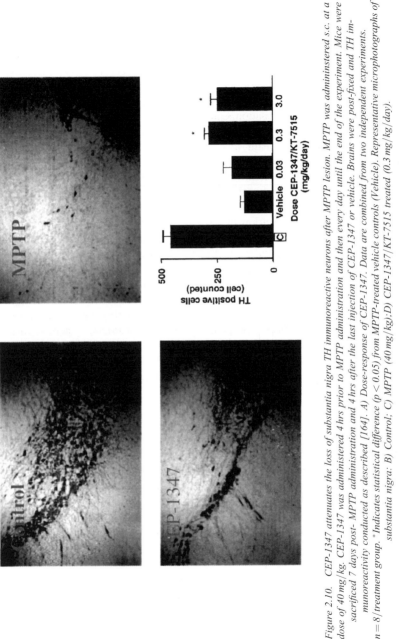

*Figure 2.10. CEP-1347 attenuates the loss of substantia nigra TH immunoreactive neurons after MPTP lesion. MPTP was administered s.c. at a dose of 40 mg/kg. CEP-1347 was administered 4 hrs prior to MPTP administration and then every day until the end of the experiment. Mice were sacrificed 7 days post-MPTP administration and 4 hrs after the last injection of CEP-1347 or vehicle. Brains were post-fixed and TH immunoreactivity conducted as described [164]. A) Dose-response of CEP-1347. Data are combined from two independent experiments. n = 8/treatment group. *Indicates statistical difference (p < 0.05) from MPTP-treated vehicle controls (Vehicle). Representative microphotographs of substantia nigra: B) Control; C) MPTP (40 mg/kg); D) CEP-1347/KT-7515 treated (0.3 mg/kg/day).*

NBM lesion model (see section 5.5), suggesting a common mechanism of neuroprotection between these models.

### 5.5.2 Neuroprotective Activity of CEP-1347 in MPTP-Treated Non-Human Primates

The neuroprotective activity of CEP-1347 in MPTP-treated mice was extended to a more relevant non-human primate MPTP model. MPTP-treated primates display behavioral impairments that closely resemble locomotor deficits seen in human Parkinson's disease including bradykinesia, postural instability, gait disturbances and tremor [139,145]. The primate model utilized for evaluation of CEP-1347 efficacy entailed the weekly administration of a low dose of MPTP to mimic the slowly progressing dopaminergic loss and behavioral impairment of PD [145]. In these studies, CEP-1347 was administered systemically prior to and during the MPTP treatments to assess the effects of this compound on MPTP-induced locomotor deficits and immunohistochemical parameters.

CEP-1347 administration (1 mg/kg/day) significantly attenuated the MPTP-mediated decline in behavioral deficits, which included bradykinesia, gait disturbances, tremor and postural instability [165]. Moreover, CEP-1347 significantly attenuated MPTP-induced deficits in global motor activity as assessed by activity monitors that were continuously attached to the animals (*Figure 2.11*) [165]. Post-mortem analysis revealed that CEP-1347 administration significantly reduced the MPTP-mediated loss of TH-positive neurons in the substantia nigra and that the behavioral attenuation was associated with the neuroprotective sparing of these neurons.

### 5.5.3 CEP-1347 Inhibition of MPTP-Mediated Activation of the JNK Signaling Pathway

Activation of the JNK signaling pathway leads to apoptotic neuronal death in various cell culture models of neurodegeneration (see Section 2). The activation of the JNK pathway was studied in MPTP-treated mice by using antibodies directed against the phospho-specific epitopes of JNK and its upstream regulatory kinase MKK4 (also known as JNKK, SEK1). A single peripheral MPTP injection to mice evoked an increase in levels of phosphorylated MKK4 and its downstream substrate, JNK, in the substantia nigra and increased the levels of phosphorylated MKK4 (but not phospho-JNK) in the striatum [166]. The maximal elevation of phospho-kinases occurred within hours of administration and simultaneously with formation of $MPP^+$ in the CNS. The $MPP^+$ mediated inhibition of mitochondrial respiration also occurs simultaneously with formation of $MPP^+$ in the CNS [167–169]. The close temporal correlation between $MPP^+$-mediated inhibition of mitochon-

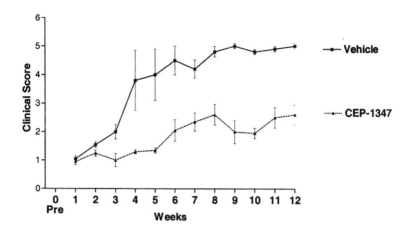

Laval University Disability Scale for MPTP Monkeys

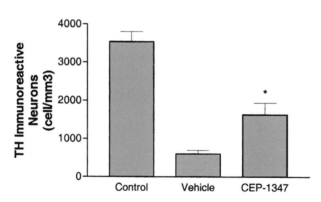

*Figure 2.11. CEP-1347 administration attenuates MPTP-induced locomotor deficits and loss of TH + neurons in MPTP treated cynomolgus monkeys. Fourteen cynomologous monkeys were gradually exposed to MPTP at a single weekly dose of 0.5 mg/kg s.c. for 10 weeks or until they reached a behavioral endpoint. Eight of the animals were administered CEP-1347 as a single s.c. daily dose of 1 mg/kg, and six animals were administered vehicle injections beginning two weeks prior to the initial MPTP dose. A) CEP-1347 significantly attenuated MPTP-mediated increase in parkinsonism; B) CEP-1347 significantly attenuated the MPTP-mediated decline in TH + neurons in the substantia nigra.*

drial function and the activation of both MKK4 and JNK pathway indicated there existed a relationship between these two events. The exact biochemical events that couple MPP$^+$ inhibition to activation of these kinases is not known.

This finding of MPTP-mediated MKK4 and JNK phosphorylation demonstrated that activation of this kinase pathway could be measured *in vivo* in the CNS, and that a known neurotoxin, with relevance to Parkinson's disease, could activate this pathway.

CEP-1347 was assessed for its ability to inhibit activation of this pathway in MPTP-treated mice (*Figure 2.12*). A single systemic administration of CEP-1347, at doses that attenuate neurodegeneration *in vivo* (including MPTP-induced neurodegeneration) inhibited the MPTP-mediated phosphorylation of both MKK4 and JNK [166]. Since these kinases are involved in stress-induced apoptotic death in a number of systems, the data implicate the JNK/SAPK kinase-signaling pathway in MPTP-induced dopaminergic degeneration.

### 5.5.4 CEP-1347 Does Not Affect Events Associated with MPTP Neurotoxicity

Exposure to MPTP or other similar environmental neurotoxins are unlikely to be a cause of the vast majority of cases of idiopathic PD. Thus neuroprotective activities that result from inhibition of MAO-B or inhibit MPP+ uptake into dopaminergic terminals would be considered ancillary activities that would manifest themselves as false positive neuroprotective activities and would confound any neuroprotective activity produced by inhibition of a kinase involved in the cell death process [170,171]. As such, CEP-1347 has been extensively characterized for its effect on MPTP toxicity at the level of monoamine oxidase inhibition, dopamine uptake and for interfering with MPP$^+$ inhibition of mitochondrial respiration.

*In vitro*, CEP-1347 did not inhibit monoamine oxidase B or dopamine uptake in brain homogenates or in functional isolated synaptosomes, respectively [164]. More recently, CEP-1347 was found not to inhibit the formation of MPP$^+$ in the CNS indicating that it did not affect MAO-B *in vivo*. These data support the *in vitro* data that CEP-1347 did not elicit its neuroprotective activity at the level of inhibition of MPTP metabolism or MPP$^+$ uptake into dopaminergic neurons.

The ability of CEP-1347 to affect MPP$^+$ inhibition of mitochondrial function *in vitro* (in striatal brain slices) and *in vivo* was also assessed. A consequence of inhibition of mitochondrial complex I is an increase in glycolysis with a significant increase in cellular lactate production [172,173]. CEP-1347, at doses that are neuroprotective and that inhibit kinase phosphorylation, did not affect MPTP (MPP$^+$)-mediated increases in lactate levels in striatal brain

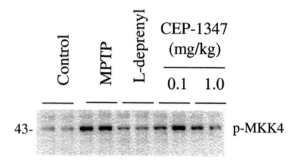

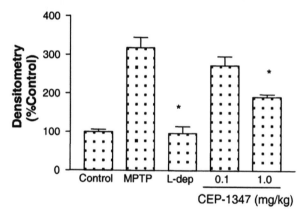

*Figure 2.12. CEP-1347 administration inhibits MPTP-mediated increases in phospho-MKK4 levels in the substantia nigra. L-deprenyl (2.5 mg/kg/injection;ip) was pre-administered to mice 18 and 2 hrs prior to MPTP administration. CEP-1347 (0.1 and 1.0 mg/kg) was administered 4 hrs prior to MPTP administration. Midbrain (containing the substantia nigra) were removed four hrs after MPTP administration and assessed for phospho-MKK4 levels. A) phospho-MKK4 immunoblot, D) phospho-MKK4 graphical representation. For the graphs, data are from two experiments, values are averages ± SEM, n = 5 per group. \*Indicates statistically different from MPTP-treated vehicle control.*

slices or in the striatum of mice, indicating that the CEP-1347 site of action lies downstream of MPP$^+$ inhibition of mitochondrial function. This observation is consistent with the hypothesis that CEP-1347 is neuroprotective in these models by inhibiting a kinase that lies within the JNK signaling cascade.

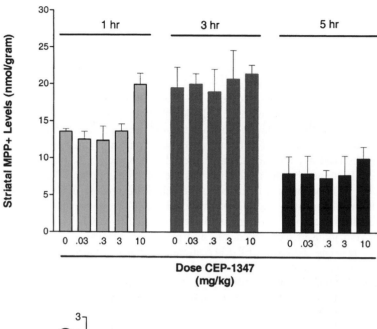

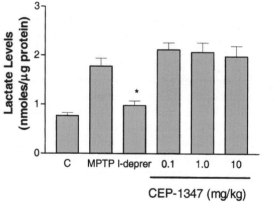

*Figure 2.13.   CEP-1347 does not affect striatal levels of MPP + or MPP + -mediated increases in striatal lactate levels. A. MPP + brain levels were assessed in the striatum 1, 3 and 5 hrs after dosing, in the presence of increasing doses of CEP-1347. CEP-1347 administration did not affect levels of MPP + in the striata. B. Striata from the experiment described in Figure 2.4 were assessed for lactate levels. MPTP administration increased striatal lactate by approximately 2-fold. CEP-1347 administration did not affect MPTP-mediated increases in striatal lactate, indictating that CEP-1347 does not affect MPP + inhibition of mitochondrial function.*

## 5.6 RESCUE OF HEARING LOSS

More than one-third of the aging population will suffer from substantial hearing loss. In the majority of cases the loss of hearing in an individual results from death of hair cells in the organ of Corti, the auditory organ. Because hair cells do not regenerate in the mammalian cochlea, the loss, whether caused by noise or toxins, is irreversible. Apoptosis as measured by DNA fragmentation has been identified in auditory hair cell death after ototoxic and intense noise trauma [174]. Based on immunohistochemistry, the apoptotic pathway involves JNK activation. Phospho-JNK and phospho-c-Jun immunoreactive hair cells were observed in cochlear explants exposed to neomycin. The only part of the hair cells stained by the antibodies was the nuclei, supporting the hypothesis that the JNK pathway is involved in the cell death process. Based on the potential involvement of the JNK pathway, CEP-1347 was evaluated for survival effects in the cochlea. In organotypic cochlear cultures CEP-1347 prevented neomycin induced hair cell death, and promoted survival of dissociated cochlear neurons. *In vivo*, CEP-1347 attenuated noise-induced hearing loss in guinea pigs. The protective effect was demonstrated by functional tests showing a lower hearing threshold shift in CEP-1347-treated than non-treated animals, and by morphological assessment showing less hair cell death in CEP-1347-treated cochlea [174].

## 5.7 SUMMARY

CEP-1347, a semi-synthetic derivative of the natural product K-252a, is a potent, selective inhibitor of the cJun-amino terminal kinase pathway currently under clinical evaluation for the treatment of neurodegenerative diseases. The molecular target(s) of CEP-1347 affecting the JNK pathway remain under investigation, however, a candidate responsible for the survival promoting effects appear to be the multiple lineage kinase family members. CEP-1347 is a potent inhibitor of the MLK family, while it does not inhibit MEKK1 activated JNK1 in cells.

The activity of CEP-1347 in three models of neurodegeneration is described. The neuroprotective activity of CEP-1347 occurs with peripheral administration within the same efficacious dose range (see *Table 2.4*) suggesting that similar mechanistic features participate in the degeneration of these neurons. The neuroprotective activity of CEP-1347 is independent of the type of neuronal injury. As described, CEP-1347 prevents neuronal degeneration after excitotoxic injury, mechanical transection or mitochondrial inhibition. In the MPTP model of mitochondrial inhibition, the JNK signaling cascade is activated and inhibited by CEP-1347 administration at the same efficacious dose range. These data

Table 2.4.   EFFICACIOUS DOSE-RANGES FOR CEP-1347 IN ANIMAL MODELS
OF NEURODEGENERATION[a]

| Animal Model | Marker | Efficacious Doses (mg/kg/dose) | Reference |
|---|---|---|---|
| NBM Lesion Model | Cortical ChAT Enzyme Activity (cholinergic terminals) | 0.03–1.0 mg/kg/dose | 116 |
| NBM Lesion Model | NBM ChAT cell bodies | 0.03 mg/kg/dose | 116 |
| NBM Lesion Model | Cognitive attentional behavior | 0.03 mg/kg/dose | 129 |
| Fimbria-Fornix Lesion Model | ChAT immunoreactive cell number | 1.0 mg/kg/dose | 133 |
| Fimbria-Fornix Lesion Model | Hippocampal ChAT enzyme activity | 0.25 mg/kg/day[b] | 133 |
| MPTP (low dose)[c] | Striatal dopaminergic terminals | 0.1–3.0 mg/kg/dose | 164 |
| MPTP (high dose)[d] | TH$^+$ cell body number | 0.3–3.0 mg/kg | 166 |

[a]CEP-1347 was dosed subcutaneous on a daily basis unless otherwise indicated.
[b]CEP-1347 infused via subcutaneous implanted osmotic minipump at indicated daily dose.
[c]MPTP administered at a dose of 20 mg/kg.
[d]MPTP administered at a dose of 40 mg/kg.
[e]Measurements made 4 hrs after MPTP injection, single CEP-1347 dose.

indicate that in these models of selected neuronal degeneration, a similar neurodegenerative pathway may be activated (the JNK signaling cascade) and that
this pathway participates in the neurodegenerative process in these neurons.
Based on its mechanism, CEP-1347 may prevent degeneration in a wide-range
of neurodegenerative diseases and is currently under clinical evaluation.

## ACKNOWLEDGEMENTS

The authors would like to acknowledge the support and contributions from
many scientists and collaborators that have contributed to this project. Speci-
fically, we would like to acknowledge the accomplishments of Chikara
Murakata, Yuzuru Matsuda, Masami Kaneko, Nicola T. Neff, Craig A. Dionne,
Donna Bozyczko-Coyne, Ernest Knight Jr., James C. Kauer, Mark Ator,
Thelma S. Angeles, Mathew Miller, Mary Savage, Marcie A. Glicksman, John
P. Mallamo, Rick Scott, and Jeffry Vaught.

# REFERENCES

1   Thompson, C. B. Apoptosis in the pathogenesis and treatment of disease. *Science* 1995, *267*, 1456–1462.

2   Johnson, E. M.; Deckwerth, T. L., Deshmukh, M. Neuronal death in developmental models: possible implications in neuropathology. *Brain Pathology* 1996, *6*, 397–409.

3   Oppenheim, R. W. Cell death during development of the nervous system. *Ann. Rev. Neurosci.* 1991, *14*, 453–501.

4   Honig, L. S.; Rosenburg, R. N. Apoptosis and neurological disease. *Am. J. Med.* 2000, *108*, 317–330.

5   Bergeron, L.; Yuan, J. Sealing one's fate: control of cell death in neurons *Curr. Opin. Neurobiol.* 1998, *8*, 55–63.

6   Smale, G.; Nichols, N. R.; Brady, D. R.; Finch, C. E.; Horton, Jr. W. E. Evidence for apoptotic cell death in Alzheimer's disease. *Exp. Neurol.* 1995, *133*, 225–230.

7   Li, W. P.; Chan, W. Y.; Lai, H. W. L.; Yew, D. T. Terminal dUTP Nick End Labeling (TUNEL) positive cells in the different regions of the brain in normal aging and Alzheimer patients. *J. Mol. Neurosci.* 1997, *8*, 75–82.

8   Mielke, K.; Herdegen, T. JNK and p38 stresskinases – degenerative effectors of signal-transduction-cascades in the nervous system. *Prog. Neurobiol.* 2000, *61*, 45–60.

9   Estus, S.; Zaks, W. J.; Freeman, R. S.; Gruda, M.; Bravo, R.; Johnson, E. M. Altered gene expression in neurons during programmed cell death: Identification of c-Jun as necessary for neuronal apoptosis. *J. Cell. Biol.* 1999, *127*, 1717–1727.

10  Schlingensiepen, K. H.; Wallnik, F.; Kunst, M.; Schlingensiepen, R.; Herdengen, T.; Brysch, W. The role of Jun transcription factor expression and phosphorylation in neuronal differentiation, neuronal cell death, and plastic adaptations *in vivo. Cell. Mol. Neurobiol.* 1994, *14*, 487–505.

11  Ham, J.; Babij, C.; Whitfield, J.; Pfarr, C. M.; Lallemand, D.; Yaniv, M.; and Rubin, L. L. A c-Jun dominant negative mutant protects sympathetic neurons against programmed cell death. *Neuron* 1995, *14*, 927–939.

12  Hibi, M.; Lin, A.; Smeal, T.; Minden, A.; Karin, M. Identification of an oncoprotein- and UV-responsive protein kinase that binds and potentiates the c-jun activation domain. *Genes Dev.* 1993, *7*, 2135–2148.

13  Dérijard, B.; Hibi, M.; Wu, I-H.; Barrett, T.; Su, B.; Deng, T.; Karin, M.; Davis, R. J. JNK1: A protein kinase stimulated by UV light and Ha-Ras that binds and phosphorylates the c-Jun activation domain. *Cell* 1994, *76*, 1025–1037.

14  Kyriakis, J. M.; Banerjee, P.; Nikolakaki, E.; Dal, T.; Rubie, E. A.; Ahmad, M. F.; Avruch, J.; Woodgett, J. R. The stress-activated protein kinase subfamily of c-Jun kinases. *Nature* 1994, *369*, 156–160.

15  Watson, A.; Eilers, A.; Lallemand, D.; Kyriakis, J.; Rubin, L. L.; Ham, J. Phosphorylation of c-Jun is necessary for apoptosis induced by survival signal withdrawal in cerebellar granule neurons. *J. Neurosci.* 1998, *18*, 751–762.

16  Le-Niculescu, H.; Bonfoco, E.; Kasuya, Y.; Claret, F. X.; Green, D. R.; Karin, M. Withdrawal of survival factors results in activation of the JNK pathway in neuronal cells leading to Fas ligand induction and cell death. *Mol. Cell. Biol.* 1999, *19*, 751–763.

17  Deijard, B.; Raingeaud, J.; Barrett, T.; Wu, I. H.; Han, J.; Ulevitch, R. J.; Davis, R. J. Independent human MAP-kinase signal transduction pathways defined by MEK and MKK isoforms. *Science* 1995, *267*, 682–685.

18  Sanchez, I.; Hughes, R. T.; Mayer, B. J.; Yee, K.; Woodgett, J. R.; Avruch, J.; Kyriakis, J. M.; Zon, L. I. Role of SAPK/ERK kinase-1 in the stress-activated pathway regulating transcription factor c-Jun. *Nature* 1994, *372*, 794–798.

19  Lin, A.; Minden, A.; Martinetto, H.; Claret, F. X.; Lange-Carter, C.; Mercurio, F.; Johnson, G.
    L.; Karin, M. Identification of a dual specificity kinase that activates the Jun kinases and p38-
    Mpk2. *Science* 1995, *268*, 286–290.

20  Lawler, S.; Cuenda, A.; Goedert, M.; Cohen, P. SKK4, a novel activator of stress-activated
    protein kinase-1 (SAPK1/JNK). *FEBS Lett.* 1997, *414*, 153–158.

21  Lu, X.; Nemoto, S.; Lin, A. Identification of c-Jun NH2-terminal protein kinase (JNK)-acti-
    vating kinase 2 as an activator of JNK but not p38. *J. Biol. Chem.* 1997, *272*, 24751–24754.

22  Tournier, C.; Whitmarsh, A.; Cavanagh, J.; Barrett, T., Davis, R. Mitogen-activated protein
    kinase kinase 7 is an activator of the c-Jun NH2-terminal kinase. *Proc. Natl. Acad. Sci.*, *USA*
    1997, *94*, 7737–7342.

23  Wu, A.; Wu, J.; Jacinto, E.; Karin, M. Molecular cloning and characterization of human
    JNKK2, a novel Jun NH2-terminal kinase-specific kinase. *Mol. Cell. Biol.* 1997, *17*, 7407–
    7416.

24  Foltz, I. N.; Gerl, R. E.; Wieler, J. S.; Lyckach, M.; Salmon, R. A.; Schrader, J. W. Human
    mitogen-activated protein kinase kinase 7 (MKK7) is a highly conserved c-Jun N-terminal
    kinase/stress-activated protein kinase (JNK/SAPK) activated by environmental stresses and
    physiological stimuli. *J. Biol. Chem.* 1998, *273*, 9344–9351.

25  Tibbles, L. A.; Woodgett, J. R. The stress-activated protein kinase pathways. *Cell. Mol. Life.
    Sci.* 1998, *55*, 1230–1254.

26  Xia, Z.; Dickens, M.; Raingeaud, J.; Davis, R. J.; Greenberg, M. E. Opposing effects of ERK
    and JNK-p38 MAP kinases on apoptosis. *Science* 1995, *270*, 1326–1331.

27  Kanamoto, T.; Mota, M.; Takefa, K.; Rubin, L.; Miyazono, K.; Ichijo, H.; Bazenet, C. Role of
    apoptosis signal-regulating kinase in regulation of the c-Jun N-terminal kinase pathway and
    apoptosis in sympathetic neurons. *Mol. Cell. Biol.* 2000, *20*, 196–204.

28  Teramoto, H.; Coso, O. A.; Miyata, H.; Igishi, T.; Miki, T.; Gutkind, J. S. Signaling from the
    small GTP-binding proteins Rac1 and Cdc42 to the c-Jun N-terminal kinase/stress-activated
    protein kinase pathway. A role for mixed lineage kinase 3/protein tyrosine kinase 1, a novel
    member of the mixed lineage kinase family. *J. Biol. Chem.* 1996, *271*, 27225–27228.

29  Bazenet, C. E.; Mota, M. A.; Rubin, L. L. The small GTP-binding protein Cdc42 is required
    for nerve growth factor withdrawal-induced neuronal death.*Proc. Natl. Acad. Sci.,USA* 1998,
    *95*, 3984–3989.

30  Yang, D. D.; Kuan, C. Y.; Whitmarsh, A. J.; Rincón M.; Zheng, T. S.; Davis, R. J.; Rakic, P.;
    Flavell, R. A. Absence of excitotoxicity-induced apoptosis in the hippocampus of mice lacking
    the Jnk3 gene. *Nature* 1997, *389*, 865–870.

31  Behrens, A.; Sibilia, M.; Wagner, E. F. Amino-terminal phosphorylation of c-Jun regulates
    stress-induced apoptosis and cellular proliferation. *Nature Genetics* 1999, *21*, 326–329.

32  Brecht, S.; Gass, P.; Anton, F.; Bravo, R.; Zimmermann, M.; Herdegen, T. Induction of c-Jun
    and suppression of CREB transcription factor proteins in axotomized neurons of substantia
    nigra and covariation with tyrosine hydroxylase. *Mol. Cell. Neurosci.* 1994, *5*, 431–441.

33  Brecht, S.; Martin-Villalba, A.; Zuschratter, W.; Bravo, B.; Herdegen, T. Transection of rat
    fimbria-fornix induces lasting expression of c-Jun protein in axotomized septal neurons im-
    munonegative for choline acetyltransferase and nitric oxide synthase. *Experimental Neurology*
    1995, *134*, 112–125.

34  Ferrer, I.; Pozas, E.; Ballabriga, J.; Planas, A. M. Strong c-Jun/AP-1 immunoreactivity is
    restricted to apoptotic cells following intracerebral ibotenic acid injection in developing rats.
    *Neurosci. Res.* 1997, *28*, 21–31.

35  Jenkins, R.; O'Shea, R.; Thomas, K. L.; Hunt, S. P. c-Jun expression in substantia nigra
    neurons following striatal 6-hydroxydopamine lesions in the rat. *Neurosci.* 1993, *53*,
    447–455.

36  Butterworth, N. J.; Dragunow, M. Medial septal cholinergic neurons express c-Jun but do not
    undergo DNA fragmentation after fornix-fimbria transections. *Mol. Brain Res.* 1996, *43*, 1–12.

37  Leah, J. D.; Herdegen, T.; Bravo, R. Selective expression of Jun proteins following axotomy and axonal-transport block in peripheral nerves in the rat- evidence for a role in the regeneration process. *Brain Res.* 1991, *566*, 198–207.

38  Defelipe, C.; Hunt, S. P. The differential control of c-Jun expression in regenerating sensory neurons and their association with glial cells. *J. Neurosci.* 1994, *14*, 2911–2923.

39  Draganow, M.; Beilharz, E.; Sirimane, E.; Lawlor, P.; Williams, C.; Brave, R; Gluckman, P. Immediate-early gene protein expression in neurons undergoing delayed death, but not necrosis, following hypoxic-ischemic injury to the young rat brain. *Mol. Brain Res.*, 1994, *25*, 19–33.

40  Mielke, K.; Brecht, S.; Dorst, A.; Herdegen, T. Activity and expression of JNK1, p38 and ERK kinases, c-Jun N-terminal phosphorylation, and c-jun promoter binding in the adult rat brain following kainate-induced seizures. *Neuroscience* 1999, *91*, 471–483.

41  Herdegen, T.; Claret, F. X.; Kallunli, T.; Martin-Villalba, A.; Winter, C.; Hunter, T.; Karin, M. Lasting N-terminal phosphorylation of c-Jun and activation of c-Jun N-terminal kinases after neuronal injury. *J. Neurosci.* 1998, *18*, 5124–5135.

42  Roffler-Tarlov, S.; Brown, J. J.; Tarlov, E.; Stolarov, J.; Chapman, D. L.; Alexiou, M.; Papaioannou, V. E. Programmed cell death in the absence of c-Fos and c-Jun. *Development* 1996, *122*, 1–9.

43  Dong, C.; Yang, D. D.; Wysk, M.; Whitmarsh, A. J.; Davis, R. J.; Flavell, R. A. Defective T cell differentiation in the absence of Jnk1. *Science* 1998, *282*, 2092–2095.

44  Yang, D. D.; Conze, D.; Whitmarsh, A. J.; Barrett, T.; Davis, R. J.; Rincon, M.; Flavell, R. A. Differentiation of CD4 + T cells to Th1 cells requires MAP kinase JNK2. *Immunity* 1998, *9*, 575–585.

45  Kuan, C. Y.; Yang, D. D.; Samanta, D. R.; Davis, R. J.; Rakic, P.; Flavell, R. A. The Jnk1 and Jnk2 protein kinases are required for regional specific apoptosis during early brain development. *Neuron* 1999, *22*, 667–676.

46  Anderson, A. J.; Su, J. H.; Cotman, C. W. DNA damage and apoptosis in Alzheimer's disease: Colocalization with c-Jun immunoreactivity, relationship to brain area, and effect of postmortem delay. *J. Neurosci.* 1996, *16*, 1710–1719.

47  Reynolds, C. H.; Utton, M. A.; Gibb, G. M.; Yates, A.; Anderton, B. H. Stress-activated protein kinase/c-Jun N-terminal kinase phosphorylates $\tau$ protein. *J. Neurochem.* 1997, *68*, 1736–1744.

48  Kase, H.; Iwahashi, K.; Matsuda, Y. K-252a, A potent inhibitor of protein kinase C from microbial origin. *J. Antibiot.* (Tokyo) 1986, *39*, 1059–1065.

49  Kase, H.; Iwahashi, K.; Nakanishi, S.; Matsuda, Y.; Yamada, K.; Takahashi, M.; Murakata, C.; Sato, A.; Kaneko, M. K-252 compounds, novel and potent inhibitors of protein kinase C and cyclic nucleotide-dependent protein kinases. *Biochem. Biophys. Res. Commun.* 1987, *142*, 436–440.

50  Knusel, B.; Hefti, F. K-252 compounds: modulators of neurotrophic signal transduction. *J. Neurochem.* 1992, *59*, 1987–1996.

51  Maroney, A. C.; Lipfert, L.; Forbes, M. E.; Glicksman, M. A.; Neff, N. T.; Siman, R.; Dionne, C. A. K-252a induces tyrosine phosphorylation of the focal adhesion kinase and neurite outgrowth in human neuroblastoma SH-SY5Y cells. *J. Neurochem.* 1995, *64*, 540–549.

52  Borasio, G. D. Differential effects of the protein kinase inhibitor K-252a on the *in vitro* survival of chick embryonic neurons. *Neurosci. Lett.* 1990, *108*, 207–212.

53  Glicksman, M. A.; Prantner, J. E.; Meyer, S. L.; Forbes, M. E.; Dasgupta, M.; Lewis, M. E.; Neff, N. T. K-252a and staurosporine promote choline acetyltransferase activity in rat spinal cord culture. *J. Neurochem.* 1993, *61*, 210–221.

54  Glicksman, M. A.; Forbes, M. E.; Prantner, J. E.; Neff, N. T. K-252a promotes survival and choline acetyltransferase activity in striatal and basal forebrain neuronal cultures. *J. Neurochem.* 1995, *64*, 1502–1512.

55  Cheng, B.; Barger, S. W.; Mattson, M. P. Staurosporine, K-252a and K-252b stabilize calcium homeostasis and promote survival of CNS neurons in the absence of glucose. *J. Neurochem.* 1994, *62*, 1319–1329.

56  Goodman, Y.; Mattson, M. P. Staurosporine and K-252a compounds protect hippocampal neurons against amyloid β-peptide toxicity and oxidative injury. *Brain Res.* 1994, *650*, 170–174.

57  Rotella, D. P.; Glicksman, M. A.; Pranter, J. E.; Neff, N. T.; Hudkins, R. L. The effect of pyrrolo[3,4-c]carbazole derivatives on spinal cord ChAT activity. *Bioorg. Med. Chem. Lett.* 1995, *5*, 1167–1171.

58  Matsuda, Y.; Fukuda, J. Inhibition by K-252a, a new inhibitor of protein kinase, of nerve growth factor-induced neurite outgrowth of chick embryo dorsal root ganglion cells. *J. Neurosci. Lett.* 1988, *87*, 11–17.

59  Hashimoto, S. K-252a, a potent protein kinase inhibitor, blocks nerve growth factor-induced neurite outgrowth and changes in the phosphorylation of proteins in PC12 cells. *J. Cell Biol.* 1988, *107*, 1531–1539.

60  Berg, M. M.; Sternberg, D. W.; Parada, L. F.; Chao, M. V. K-252a inhibits nerve growth factor-induced trk proto-oncogene tyrosine phosphorylation and kinase activity. *J. Biol. Chem.* 1992, *267*, 13–16.

61  Tapley, P.; Lamballe, F.; Barbacid, M. K-252a is a selective inhibitor of the tyrosine protein kinase activity of the trk family of oncogenes and neurotrophin receptors. *Oncogene* 1992, *7*, 371–381.

62  Ohmichi, M.; Decker, S. J.; Pang, I.; Saltiel, A. R. Inhibition of the cellular actions of nerve growth factor by staurosporine and K-252a results from the attenuation of the activity of the trk tyrosine kinase. *Biochemistry* 1992, *31*, 4034–4039.

63  Muroya, K.; Hashimoto, Y.; Hattori, S.; Nakamuru, S. Specific inhibition of NGF receptor tyrosine kinase activity by K-252a. *Biochim. Biophys. Acta.* 1992, *1135*, 353–356.

64  Nye, S. H.; Squinto, S. P.; Glass, D. J.; Stitt, T. N.; Hantzopoulos, P.; Macchi, M. J.; Lindsaay, N. S.; Ip, N. Y.; Yancopoulos, G. D. K-252a and staurosporine selectively block autophosphorylation of neurotrophin receptors and neurotrophin-mediated responses. *Mol. Biol. Cell* 1992, *3*, 677–686.

65  Kaneko, M.; Saito, Y.; Saito, H.; Matsumoto, T.; Matsuda, Y.; Vaught, J. L.; Dionne, C. A.; Angeles, T. A.; Glicksman, M. A.; Neff, N. T.; Rotella, D. P.; Kauer, J. C.; Mallamo, J. P.; Hudkins, R. L.; Murakata, C. Neurotrophic 3,9-Alkylthiomethyl- and -Alkoxymethyl-K-252a derivatives. *J. Med. Chem.* 1997, *40*, 1863–1869.

66  Angeles, T. S.; Steffler, C.; Bartlett, B. A.; Hudkins, R. L.; Stephens, R. M.; Kaplan, D. R.; Dionne, C. A. Enzyme linked immunosorbant assay for Trk A tyrosine kinase activity. *Anal. Biochem.* 1996, *236*, 49–55.

67  Kase, H.; Iwahashi, K.; Nakanishi, S.; Matsuda, Y.; Yamada, K.; Takahashi, M.; Murakata, C.; Sato, A.; Kaneko, M. K-252 compounds, novel and potent inhibitors of protein kinase C and cyclic nucleotide-dependent protein kinases. *Biochem. Biophys. Res. Commun.* 1987, *142*, 436–440.

68  Borasio, G. D.; Hostmann, S.; Anneser, J. M. H.; Neff, N. T.; Glicksman, M. A. CEP-1347/KT7515, a JNK pathway inhibitor supports the in vitro survival of chick embryonic neurons. *NeuroReport* 1998, *9*, 1435–1439.

69  Maroney, A. C.; Glicksman, M. A.; Basma, A. N.; Walton, K. M.; Knight Jr., E.; Murphy, C. A.; Bartlett, B. A.; Finn, J. P.; Angeles, T.; Matsuda, Y.; Neff, N. T.; Dionne, C. A. Motoneuron apoptosis is blocked by CEP-1347 (KT-7515), a novel inhibitor of the JNK signaling pathway. *J. Neurosci.* 1998 *18*, 104–111.

70  Comella, J. X.; Sanz-Rodriguez, C.; Aldea, M.; Esquerda, J. E. Skeletal muscle-derived trophic factors prevent motoneurons from entering an active cell death program *in vitro. J. Neurosci.* 1994, *14*, 2674–2686.

71   Milligan, C. E.; . Oppenheim, R. W.; Schwartz, L. M. Motoneurons deprived of trophic support *in vitro* require new gene expression to undergo programmed cell death *J. Neurobiol.* 1994, *25*, 1005–1016.

72   Arakawa, Y.; Sendtner, M.; Thoenen, H. Survival effect of ciliary neurotrophic factor (CNTF) on chick embryonic motoneurons in culture: Comparison with other neurotrophic factors and cytokines *J. Neurosci.* 1990, *10*, 3507–3515.

73   Hughes, R. A.; Sendtner, M.; Thoenen, H. Members of several gene families influence survival of rat motoneurons *in vitro* and *in vivo. J. Neurosci. Res.* 1993, *36*, 663–671.

74   Henderson, C. E.; Camu, W.; Mettling, C.; Gouin, A.; Poulsen, K.; Karihaloo, M.; Rullamas, J.; Evans, T.; McMahon, S. B.; Armaini, M. P.; Berkemeier, L.; Phillips, H. S.; Rosenthal, A. Neurotrophins promote motor neuron survival and are present in embryonic limb bud. *Nature* 1993, *363*, 266–270.

75   Henderson, C. E.; Phillips, H. S.; Pollock, R. A.; Davies, A. M.; Lemeulle, C.; Armanini, M.; Simpson, L. C.; Moffet, B.; Vandlen, R. A.; Koliatsos, V. E.; Rosenthal, A. GDNF: A potent survival factor for motoneurons present in peripheral nerve and muscle. *Science* 1994, *266*, 1062–1064.

76   Maroney, A. C.; Glicksman, M. A.; Basma, A. N.; Walton, K. M.; Knight, E.; Murphy, C. A.; Bartlett, B. A.; Finn, J. P.; Angeles, T.; Matsuda, Y.; Neff, N. T.; Dionne, C. A. motoneuron apoptosis is blocked by CEP-1347, a novel inhibitor of the JNK signaling pathway. *J. Neurosci.* 1998, *18*, 104–111.

77   Rosette, C.; Karin, M. Ultraviolet light and osmotic stress: Activation of the JNK cascade through multiple growth factor and cytokine receptors. *Science* 1996, *274*, 1194–1197.

78   Zanke, B. W.; Boudreau, K.; Rubie, E.; Winnett, E.; Tibbles, L. A.; Zon, L.; Kyriakis, J.; Liu, F-F; Woodgett, J. R. The stress-activated protein kinase pathway mediates cell death following injury induced by *cis*-platinum, UV irradiation or heat. *Current Biol.* 1996, *6*, 606–613.

79   Raingeaud, J.; Gupta, S.; Rogers, J. S.; Dickens, M.; Han, J.; Ulevitch, R. J.; Davis, R. J. Pro-inflammatory cytokines and environmental stress cause p38 mitogen-activated protein kinase activation by dual phosphorylation on tyrosine and threonine. *J. Biol. Chem.* 1996, 270, 7420–7426.

80   Rouse, J.; Cohen, P.; Trigon, S.; Morange, M.; Alonso-Llamazares, A.; Zamanillo, D.; Hunt, T.; Nebreda, A. R. A novel kinase cascade triggered by stress and heat shock that stimulates MAPKAP kinase-2 and phosphorylation of the small heat shock proteins. *Cell* 1994, *78*, 1027–1037.

81   Cuenda, A.; Rouse, J.; Doza, Y. N.; Meier, R.; Cohen, P.; Gallagher, T. F.; Young, P. R.; Lee, J. C. SB 203580 is a specific inhibitor of a MAP kinase homologue which is stimulated by cellular stresses and interleukin-1. *FEBS Lett.* 1995, *364*, 229–233.

82   Coyle, J. T.; Puttfarcken, P. Oxidative stress, glutamate, and neurodegenerative disorders. *Science* 1993, *262*, 689–694.

83   Williams, L. R. Oxidative stress, age-related neurodegeneration and the potential for neurotrophic treatment. *Cerebrovasc. Brain Metab. Rec.* 1993, *7*, 55–73.

84   Schapira, A. H. V. Oxidative stress in Parkinson's Disease. *Neuropathol. Appl. Neurobiol.* 1995, *21*, 3–9.

85   Maroney, A. C.; Finn, J. P.; Bozyczko-Coyne, D.; O'Kane, T.; Neff, N. T.; Tolkovsky, A. M.; Park, D. S.; Yan, C. Y. I.; Troy, C. M.; Greene, L. A. CEP-1347 (KT7515), an inhibitor of JNK activation, rescues sympathetic neurons and neuronally differentiated PC12 Cells from death evoked by three distinct insults. *J. Neurochem.* 1999, *73*, 1901–1912.

86   Park, D. S.; Morris, E. J.; Stefanis, L.; Troy, C. M.; Shelanski, M. L.; Geller, H. M.; Greene, L. A. Multiple pathways of neuronal death induced by DNA-damaging agents, NGF deprivation, and oxidative stress. *J. Neurosci.* 1998, *18*, 830–840.

87  Liu, Y.; Gorospe, M.; Yang, C.; Holbrook, N. J. Role of mitogen activated protein kinase phosphatase during the cellular response to genotoxic stress. *J. Biol. Chem.* 1995, *270*, 8377–8380.

88  Chen, Y. R.; Wang, X.; Templeton, D.; David, R. J.; Tan, T. H. The role of c-Jun N-terminal kinase (JNK) in apoptosis induced by ultraviolet C and γ radiation. *J. Biol. Chem.* 1996, *271*, 31929–31936.

89  Troy, C. M.; Stefanis, L.; Prochiantz, A.; Greene, L. A.; Shelanski, M. L. The contrasting roles of ICE family proteases and interleukin 1-β in apoptosis induced by trophic factor withdrawal and by copper/zinc superoxide dismutase down-regulation. *Proc. Natl. Acad. Sci. USA* 1996, *93*, 5635–5640.

90  Troy, C. M.; Stefanis, L.; Greene, L. A.; Shelanski, M. L. Mechanisms of neuronal degeneration: A final common pathway? *Neurol.* 1997, *72*, 103–111.

91  Troy, C. M.; Stefanis, L.; Greene, L. A.; Shelanski, M. L. Nedd2 is required for apoptosis after trophic factor withdrawal, but not superoxide dismutase (SOD-1) down regulation, in sympathetic neurons and PC12 cells. *J. Neurosci.* 1997, *17*, 1911–1918.

92  Green, D. R.; Scott, D. W. Activation-induced apoptosis in lymphocytes. *Curr. Opin. Immunol.* 1994, *6*, 476–487.

93  Gardner, A. M.; Johnson, G. L. Fibroblast growth factor-2 suppression of tumor necrosis factor α-mediated apoptosis requires RAS and the activation of mitogen-activated protein kinase. *J. Biol. Chem.* 1996, *271*, 14560–14566.

94  Liu, A.-G.; Hsu, H.; Goeddel, D. V.; Karin, M. Dissection of TNF receptor 1 effector functions: JNK activation is not linked to apoptosis while NF-κB activation prevents cell death. *Cell* 1996, *87*, 565–576.

95  Verheij, M.; Bose, R.; Lin, X. H.; Yao, B.; Jarvis, W. D.; Grant, S.; Birrer, M. J.; Szabo, E.; Zon, L. I.; Kyriakis, J. M.; Halmovitz-Friedman, A.; Fuks, A.; Kolesnick, R. N. Requirement for ceramide-initiated SAPK/JNK signalling in stress-induced apoptosis. *Nature* 1996, *380*, 75–79.

96  Lenczowski, J. M.; Dominguez, L.; Eder, A. M.; King, L. B.; Zacharchuk, C. M.; Ashwell, J. D. Lack of a role for Jun kinase and AP-1 in Fas-induced apoptosis. *Mol. Cell. Biol.* 1997, *17*, 170–181.

97  Faris, M.; Kokot, N.; Latinis, K.; Kasibhatla, S.; Green, D. R.; Koretzky, G. A.; Nel, A. The c-Jun N-terminal kinase cascade plays a role in stress-induced apoptosis in Jurkat cells by up-regulating Fas ligand expression. *J. Immunology* 1998, *160*, 134–144.

98  Abreu-Martin, M. T.; Palladino, A. A.; Faris, M.; Carramanzana, N. M.; Nel, A. E.; Targan, S. R. Fas activates the JNK pathway in human colonic epithelial cells: lack of a direct role in apoptosis. *Am. J. Physiol.* 1999, *276*, 599–605.

99  Glicksman, M. A.; Chiu, A. Y.; Dionne, C. A.; Kaneko, M.; Murakata, C.; Oppenheim, R. W.; Prevette, D.; Sengelaub, D. R.; Vaught, J. L.; Neff, N. T. CEP-1347/KT-7515 prevents motor neuronal programmed cell death and injury-induced dedifferentation in *vivo J. Neurobiol.* 1998, *35*, 361–370.

100  Chu-Wang, L-W.; Oppenheimer, R. W. Cell death of motor neurons in the chick embryo spinal cord. *J. Comp. Neurol.* 1978, *177*, 33–57.

101  Nordeen, E. J.; Nordeen, K. W.; Sengelaub, D. R.; Arnold, A. P. Androgens prevent normally occurring cell death in a sexually dimorphic spinal nucleus. *Science* 1985, *229*, 671–673.

102  Oppenheim, R. W. Cell death during development of the nervous system. *Ann. Rev. Neurosci.* 1991, *14*, 453–501.

103  Bartus, R. T.; Dean, R. L 3d; Beer, B.; Lippa, A. S. The cholinergic hypothesis of geriatric memory dysfunction. *Science* 1982, *217*, 408–14

104  Dunnett, S. B.; Everitt, B. J.; Robbins, T. W. The basal forebrain-cortical cholinergic system: interpreting the function consequences of excitotoxic lesions. *Trends Neurosci.* 1991, *14*, 494–501.

105    Fibiger, H. C. The organization and some projections of cholinergic neurons of the mammalian forebrain. *Brain Res. Rev.* 1982, *4*, 327–388.

106    Fibiger, H. C. Cholinergic mechanisms in learning memory and dementia: a review of recent evidence. *Trends Neurosci.* 1991, *14*, 220–223.

107    Whitehouse, P. J.; Price, D. L.; Struble, R. G.; Clark, A. W.; Delong, M. R. Alzheimer's disease and senile dementia: Loss of neurons in the basal forebrain. *Science* 1982, *215*, 237–1239.

108    Olton, D. S.; Wenk, G. L. Dementia: animal models of the cognitive impairments produced by degeneration of the basal forebrain cholinergic system. In HY Meltzer (Ed) Psychopharmacology: The Third Generation of Progress. Raven Press, New York, 1987 pp. 941–953.

109    Smith, G. Animal models of Alzheimer's disease: experimental cholinergic denervation. *Brain Res. Rev.* 1988, *13*, 103–118.

110    Bartus, R. T. On neurodegenerative diseases, models, and treatment strategies: lessons learned and lessons forgotten a generation following the cholinergic hypothesis. *Exp. Neurol.* 2000, *163*, 495–529.

111    Murray, C. L.; Fibiger, H. C. Pilocarpine and physostigmine attenuate spatial memory impairments produced by lesions of the NBM. *Behav. Neurosci.* 1986, *100*, 23–32

112    Mandel, R. J.; Gage, F. H.; Thal, L. J. Spatial learning in rats: correlation with cortical choline acetyltransferase and improvement with NGF following nbm damage. *Exp. Neurol.* 1989, *104*, 208–217.

113    Lindefors, N.; Boatel, M. L.; Mahy, N.; Persson, H. Widespread neuronal degeneration after ibotenic acid lesioning of cholinergic neurons in the nucleus basalis revealed by *in situ* hybridization. *Neurosci. Lett.* 1992, *135*, 262–264.

114    Coyle, J. T. AD: a disorder of cortical cholinergic innervation. *Science* 1983, *219*, 1184–1190.

115    Wenk, G. L.; Harrington, C. A.; Tucker, D. A.; Rance, N. E.; Walker, L. C. Basal forebrain neurons and memory: A biochemical, histological, and behavioral study of differential vulnerability to ibotenate and quisqualate. *Behav. Neurosci.* 1992, 909–923.

116    Saporito, M. S.; Brown, E. R.; Miller, M. S.; Murakata, C.; Neff, N. H.; Vaught, J. L.; Carswell, S. Preservation of cholinergic activity and prevention of neuron death by CEP-1347/KT-7515 following excitotoxic injury of the nucleus basalis magnocellularis. *Neuroscience* 1998, *86*, 461–472.

117    Carlsen, J.; Zaborszky, L.; Heimer, L. Cholinergic projections from the basal forebrain to the basolateral amygdaloid complex: A combined retrograde fluorescent and immunohistochemical study. *J. Comp. Neurol.* 1985, *234*, 155–167.

118    Mcgaughy, J.; Kaiser, T.; Sarter, M. Behavioral vigilance following infusions of 192 IgG-saporin into the basal forebrain: selectivity of the behavioral impairment and relation to cortical AChE-positive fiber density. *Behav. Neurosci.* 1996, *110*, 247–265.

119    Muir, J. L.; Dunnett, S. B.; Robbins, T. W.; Everitt, B. J. Attentional functions of the forebrain cholinergic systems: effects of intraventricular hemicholinium, physostigmine, basal forebrain lesions and intracortical grafts on a multiple-choice serial reaction time task. *Exp. Brain Res.* 1992, *89*, 611–22.

120    Muir, J. L.; Everitt, B. J.; Robbins, T. W. AMPA-induced excitotoxic lesions of the basal forebrain: a significant role for the cortical cholinergic system in attentional function. *J. Neurosci.* 1994, *14*, 2313–2326.

121    Torres, E. M.; Perry, T. A.; Blockland, A.; Wilkinson, L. S.; Wiley, R. G.; Lappi, D. A.; Dunnet, S. B. Behavioural, histochemical and biochemical consequences of selective immunolesions in discrete regions of the basal forebrain cholinergic system. *Neuroscience* 1994, *63*, 95–122.

122    Vargo, J. M.; Lai, H. V.; Marshall, J. F.; Light deprivation accelerates recovery from frontal cortical neglect: relation to locomotion and striatal Fos expression. *Behav. Neurosci.* 1998, *112*, 387–398.

123 Parasuraman, R.; Haxby, J. V. Attention and brain function in Alzheimer's Disease: a review. *Neuropsychology* 1993, *7*, 242–272.

124 Tierney, M. C.; Szalai, J; Snow, W. G.; Fisher, R. H.; Nores, A.; Nadon, G.; Dunn, E.; St George-Hyslop, P. H. Prediction of probable Alzheimer's disease in memory-impaired patients: A prospective longitudinal study. *Neurology* 1996, *46*, 661–665.

125 Dekker, A. J.; Thal, L. J. Effect of delayed treatment with nerve growth factor on choline acetyltransferase activity in the cortex of rats with lesions of the nucleus basalis magnocellularis: dose requirements. *Brain Res.* 1992, *584*, 55–63.

126 Dekker, A. J.; Winkler, J.; Ray, J.; Thal, L. J.; Gage, F. H. Grafting of nerve growth factor-producing fibroblasts reduces behavioral deficits in rats with lesions of the nucleus basalis magnocellularis. *Neuroscience*, 1994, *60*, 299–309.

127 Haroutunian, V.; Kanof, P. D.; Davis, K. L. Attenuation of nucleus basalis of Meynert lesion-induced cholinergic deficits by nerve growth factor. *Brain Res.* 1989, *487*, 200–203.

128 Hu, L.; Cote, S. L.; Cuello, C. Differential modulation of the cholinergic phenotype of the nucleus basalis magnocelluaris neurons by applying NGF at the cell body or cortical terminal fields. *Exp. Neurol.* 1997, *143*, 162–171.

129 DiCamillo, A. M.; Neff, N. T.; Carswell, S.; Haun, F. A. Chronic sparing of delayed alternation performance and choline acetyltransferase activity by CEP-1347/KT-7515 in rats with lesions of nucleus basalis magnocellularis. *Neuroscience* 1998, *86*, 473–483.

130 Dunnett, S. B.; Barth, T. M. Animal models of Alzheimer's disease and dementia (with an emphasis on cortical cholinergic systems). 1991, In *Behavioural Models in Psychopharmacology* (ed. Willner P.), pp. 359–418. Cambridge University Press, London.

131 Gage, F. H.; Armstrong, D. M.; Williams, L. R.; Varon, S. Morphological response of axotomized septal neurons to nerve growth factor. *J. Comp. Neurol.* 1988, *269*, 147–155.

132 Koliatsos, V. E.; Applegate, M. D.; Knusel, B.; Junard, E. O.; Burton, L. E.; Mobley, W. C.; Hefti, F. F.; Price, D. L. Recombinant human nerve growth factor prevents retrograde degeneration of axotomized basal forebrain cholinergic neurons in the rat. *Exp. Neurol.* 1991, *112*, 161–173.

133 Harper, S. J.; Saporito, M. S.; Hewson, L.; Young, L.; Smith, D.; Rigby, M.; Jackson, P.; Curtis, N.; Swain, C.; Hefti, F.; Vaught, J. L.; Sirinathsinghji, D.; CEP-1347 increases ChAT activity in culture and promotes cholinergic neurone survival following fimbria-fornix lesion. *Neuroreport* 2000, *11*, 2271–2276.

134 Mesulam, M. M. Human brain cholinergic pathways. *Prog. Brain Res.* 1990, *84*, 231–241.

135 Williams, L. R.; Inouye, G.; Cummins, V.; Pelleymounter, M. A. Glial cell line-derived neurotrophic factor sustains axotomized basal forebrain cholinergic neurons *in vivo*: dose-response comparison to nerve growth factor and brain-derived neurotrophic factor. *J. Pharmacol. Exp. Ther.* 1996, *277*, 1140–1151.

136 Knusel, B.; Beck, K. D.; Winslow, J.; Rosenthal, A.; Burton, L. E.; Widmer, H. R.; Nikolics, K.; Hefti, F. Brain-derived neurotrophic factor administration protects basal forebrain cholinergic but not nigral dopaminergic neurons from degenerative changes after axotomy in the adult rat brain. *J. Neurosci.* 1992, *12*, 4391–4402.

137 Hefti, F. Nerve growth factor promotes survival of septal cholinergic neurons after fimbrial transactions. *J Neurosci.* 1986, *6*, 2155–2162.

138 Agid, Y. Parkinson's disease: pathophysiology. *The Lancet* 1991, *337*, 1321–1324.

139 Langston, J. W. The etiology of Parkinson's disease with emphasis on the MPTP story.- *Neurology* 1996, *47*, S153–160.

140 Graybiel, A. M.; Hirsch, E. C.; Agid, Y. The nigrostriatal system in Parkinson's disease. *Adv. Neurol.* 1990, *53*, 17–29.

141 Jenner, P. The rationale for the use of dopamine agonists in Parkinson's disease. *Neurology* 1995, *45*, S6-12.

142   Emilien, G.; Maloteaux, J. M.; Geurts, M.; Hoogenberg, K.; Cragg, S. Dopamine receptors-physiological understanding to therapeutic intervention potential. *Pharmacol. Ther.* 1999, *84*,133–156.

143   Heikkila, R. E.; Manzino, L.; Cabbat, F. S.; Duvoisin, R. C. Protection against the dopaminergic neurotoxicity of 1-methyl-4-phenyl-1,2,3,6-tetrahydropyridine by monoamine oxidase inhibitors. *Nature* 1984, *311*, 467–469.

144   Heikkila, R. E.; Hess, A.; Duvoisin, R. C. Dopaminergic neurotoxicity of 1-methyl-4-phenyl-1,2,3,6-tetrahydropyridine in mice. *Science* 1984, *224*, 1451–1453.

145   Blanchet, P. J.; Konitsiotis, S.; Hyland, K.; Arnold, L. A.; Pettigrew, K. D.; Chase, T. N. Chronic exposure to MPTP as a primate model of progressive parkinsonism: a pilot study with a free radical scavenger. *Exp. Neurol.* 1998, *153*, 214–222.

146   Jackson-Lewis, V.; Jakowec, M.; Burke, R. E.; Przedborski, S. Time course and morphology of dopaminergic neuronal death caused by the neurotoxin 1-methyl-4-phenyl-1,2,3,6-tetrahydropyridine. *Neurodegeneration* 1995, *4*, 257–269.

147   Javitch, J. A.; D'Amato, R. J.; Strittmatter, S. M.; Snyder, S. H. Parkinsonism-inducing neurotoxin, N-methyl-4-phenyl-1,2,3,6-tetrahydropyridine: uptake of the metabolite N-methyl-4-phenylpyridine by dopamine neurons explains selective toxicity. *Proc. Natl. Acad. Sci. U.S.A.* 1985, *82*, 2173–2177.

148   Tipton, K. F; Singer, T. P. Advances in our understanding of the mechanisms of the neurotoxicity of MPTP and related compounds. *J. Neurochem.* 1993, *61*, 1191–1206.

149   Saporito, M. S.; Heikkila, R. E.; Youngster, S. K.; Nicklas, W. J.; Geller, H. M. Dopaminergic neurotoxicity of 1-methyl-4-phenylpyridinium analogs in cultured mesencephalon: relationship to dopamine uptake affinity and inhibition of mitochondrial respiration. *J. Pharmacol. Exp. Ther.* 1992, *260*, 1400–1409.

150   Nicklas, W. J.; Vyas, I.; Heikkila, R. E. Inhibition of NADH-linked oxidation in brain mitochondria by 1-methyl-4-phenylpyridine, a metabolite of the neurotoxin, 1-methyl-4-phenyl-1,2,5,6-tetrahydropyridine. *Life Sci.* 1985, *36*, 2503–2508.

151   Kindt, M. V.; Heikkila, R. E.; Nicklas, W. J. Mitochondrial and metabolic toxicity of 1-methyl-4-(2'-methylphenyl)-1,2,3,6-tetrahydropyridine. *J. Pharmacol. Exp. Ther.* 1987, *242*, 858–863.

152   Vyas, I.; Heikkila, R. E.; Nicklas, W. J. Studies on the neurotoxicity of 1-methyl-4-phenyl-1,2,3,6-tetrahydropyridine: inhibition of NAD-linked substrate oxidation by its metabolite, 1-methyl-4-phenylpyridinium. *J. Neurochem.* 1986, *46*, 1501–1507.

153   Schapira, A. H.; Gu, M.; Taanman, J. W.; Tabrisi, S. J.; Seaton, T.; Cleeter, M.; Cooper, J. M. Mitochondria in the etiology and pathogenesis of Parkinson's disease. *Ann. Neurol.* 1998,*44*, S89–98.

154   Swerdlow, R. H.; Parks, J. K.; Miller, S. W.; Tuttle, L. B.; Trimmer, P. A.; Sheehan, J. P.; Bennett, J. P. Jr.; Davis, R. E.; Parker, W. D. Jr. Origin and functional consequences of the complex I defect in Parkinson's disease. *Ann. Neurol.* 1996, *40*, 663–671.

155   Dipasquale B.; Marini A. M.; Youle R. J. Apoptosis and DNA degradation induced by 1-methyl-4-phenylpyridinium in neurons. *Biochem. Biophys. Res. Commun.* 1991, *181*, 1442–1448.

156   Hartley A.; Stone J. M.; Heron C.; Cooper J. M.; Schapira A. H. Complex I inhibitors induce dose-dependent apoptosis in PC12 cells; Relevance to Parkinson's disease. *J. Neurochem.* 1994, *63*, 1987–1990.

157   Mochizuki, H.; Nakamura, N.; Nishi, K.; Mizuno, Y. Apoptosis is induced by 1-methyl-4-phenylpyridinium ion (MPP$^+$) in ventral mesencephalic-striatal co-culture in rat. *Neurosci. Lett.* 1994, *170*, 191–194.

158   Tatton, N. A.; Kish, S. J. *In situ* detection of apoptotic nuclei in the substantia nigra compacta of 1-methyl-4-phenyl-1,2,3,6-tetrahydropyridine-treated mice using terminal deox-

ynucleotidyl transferase labelling and acridine orange staining. *Neuroscience* 1997, *77*, 1037–1048.

159 Fall, C. P.; Bennett, J. P., Jr. Characterization and time-course of MPP$^+$-induced apoptosis in numan SH-SY5Y neuroblastoma cells. *J. Neurosci. Res.* 1999, *55*, 620–628.

160 Offen, D.; Beart, P. M.; Cheung, N. S.; Pascoe, C. J.; Hocham, A.; Gorodin, S.; Melamed, E.; Bernard, R.; and Bernard, O. Transgenic mice expressing human Bcl-2 in their neurons are resistant to 6-hydroxydopamine and 1-methyl-4-phenyl-1,2,3,6-tetrahydropyridine neurotoxicity. *Proc. Natl. Acad. Sci. USA* 1998, *95*, 5789–5794.

161 Trimmer, P. A.; Smith, T. S.; Jung, A. B.; Bennett, J. P. Dopamine neurons from transgenic mice with knockout of the p53 gene resist MPTP neurotoxicity. *Neurodegeneration* 1996, *5*, 233–239.

162 Anglade, P.; Vyas, S.; Javoy-Agid, F.; Herrero, M. T.; Michel, P. P.; Marquez, J.; Mouatt-Prigent, A.; Ruberg, M.; Hirsch, E. C.; Agid, Y. Apoptosis and autophagy in nigral neurons of patients with Parkinson's disease. *Histol. Histopathol.* 1997, *12*, 25–31.

163 Hunot, S.; Brugg, B.; Ricard, D.; Michel, P. P.; Muriel, M. P.; Ruberg, M.; Faucheux, B. A.; Agid, Y.; Hirsch, E. C. Nuclear translocation of NF-KappaB is increased in dopaminergic neurons of patients with Parkinson's disease. *Proc. Natl. Acad. Sci. USA* 1997, *94*, 7531–7536

164 Saporito, M. S.; Brown, E. M.; Miller, M. S.; Carswell, S. CEP-1347/KT-7515. An inhibitior of c-jun N-terminal kinase activation attenuates the 1-methyl-4-phenyl tetrahydropyridine-mediated loss of nigrostriatal dopaminergic neurons in vivo. *J. Pharmacol. Exp. Ther.* 1999, *288*, 421–427.

165 Konitsiotis, S.; Saporito, M. S.; Flood, D. G.; Hyland, K.; Miller, M.; Lin, Y. G.; Arnold, L. A.; LePoole, K.; Bibbiani, F.; Blanchet, P. J.; Chase, T. N. The neuroprotective effects of CEP-1347 in a primate model of MPTP-induced chronic progressive parkinsonism. *Soc. Neurosci. Abst.* 1999, *25*, 1595.

166 Saporito, M. S.; Thomas, B. A.; Scott, R. W. MPTP activates c-Jun NH(2)-terminal kinase (JNK) and its upstream regulatory kinase MKK4 in nigrostriatal neurons in vivo. *J. Neurochem.* 2000, *75*, 1200–1208.

167 Rollema, H.; Johnson, E. A.; Booth, R. G.; Caldera, P.; Lampen, P.; Youngster, S. K.; Trevor, A. J.; Naiman, N.; Castagnoli, N. *In vivo* intracerebral microdialysis studies in rats of MPP$^+$ analogs and related charged species. *J. Med. Chem.* 1990, *33*, 2221–2230.

168 Cassarino, D. S.; Fall, C. P.; Swerdlow, R. H.; Smith, T. S.; Halvorsen, E. M.; Miller, S. W.; Parks, J. P.; Parker, W. D. Jr,; Bennett, J. P. Jr. Elevated reactive oxygen species and antioxidant enzyme activities in animal and cellular models of Parkinson's disease. *Biochim. Biophys. Acta.* 1997, *1362*, 77–86.

169 Chan P.; DeLanney L. E.; Irwin I.; Langston J. W.; Di Monte, D. Rapid ATP loss caused by 1-methyl-4-phenyl-1,2,3,6-tetrahydropyridine in mouse brain. *J. Neurochem.* 1991, *57*, 348–351.

170 Giovanni, A.; Sieber, B. A.; Heikkila, R. E.; Sonsalla, P. K. Correlation between the neostriatal content of the 1-methyl-4-phenylpyridinium species and dopaminergic neurotoxicity following 1-methyl-4-phenyl-1,2,3,6-tetrahydropyridine administration to several strains of mice. *J. Pharmacol. Exp. Ther.* 1991, *257*, 691–697.

171 Vaglini, F.; Fascetti, F.; Tedeschi, D.; Cavalletti, M.; Fornai, F.; Corsini, G. U. Striatal MPP+ levels do not necessarily correlate with striatal dopamine levels after MPTP treatment in mice. *Neurodegeneration* 1996, *5*, 129–136.

172 Ofori, S.; Heikkila, R. E.; Nicklas, W. J. Attenuation by dopamine uptake blockers of the inhibitory effects of 1-methyl-4-phenyl-1,2,3,6-tetrahydropyridine and some of its analogs on NADH-linked metabolism in mouse neostriatal slices. *J. Pharmacol. Exp. Ther.* 1989, *251*, 258–266.

173   Rollema, H.; Kuhr, W. G.; Kranenborg, G.; De Vries, J.; Van den Berg, C. MPP+ -induced efflux of dopamine and lactate from rat striatum have similar time courses as shown by *in vivo* brain dialysis. *J. Pharmacol. Exp. Ther.* 1988, *245*, 858–866.
174   Pirvola, U.; Xing-Quin, L.; Virkkala, J.; Murakata, C.; Camoratta, A. M.; Walton, K. W. Ylikoski, J. *J. Neurosci.* 2000, *20*, 43–50.

Progress in Medicinal Chemistry – Vol. 40,
Series Editors: F.D. King and A.W. Oxford
Guest Editors: A.B. Reitz and S.L. Dax

# 3 Discovery of Second Generation Quinazolinone Non-Nucleoside Reverse Transcriptase Inhibitors of HIV-1

JEFFREY W. CORBETT*[a] AND JAMES D. RODGERS

*DuPont Pharmaceuticals Company, Experimental Station, P. O. Box 80500,
Wilmington, DE 19880-0500, U.S.A.*

*[a]Current Address: Pharmacia Corporation, 7255-209-643, 301 Henrietta Street, Kalamazoo,
MI 49007.*

## ABSTRACT

An intensive research effort to identify potent, viable drugs for the management of acquired immunodeficiency syndrome (AIDS) resulted in the development of SUSTIVA$^{TM}$ (efavirenz), the first non-nucleoside reverse transcriptase inhibitor (NNRTI) approved by the FDA as a preferred first-line therapy. The search for NNRTIs that possess a broader activity spectrum against mutant viral forms of human immunodeficiency syndrome type-I reverse transcriptase culminated in the discovery that trifluoromethyl-containing quinazolin-2($1H$)-ones possess potent activity as non-nucleoside reverse transcriptase inhibitors (NNRTIs). This chapter reviews the discovery and structure activity relationships that resulted in the identification and subsequent preclinical and clinical development of four quinazolinone NNRTIs at the DuPont Pharmaceuticals Company.

## INTRODUCTION

### HUMAN IMMUNODEFICIENCY VIRUS

The identification of human immunodeficiency virus (HIV) and acquired immunodeficiency syndrome (AIDS) as a human health threat has spawned the search for effective pharmacological treatments and vaccines to contain and, hopefully, eradicate this devastating virus. The critical role for the discovery of effective treatments and prevention is evident in the recognition by the White House that ''serious transnational security threats emanate from pockets of Africa, including state-sponsored terrorism, drug trafficking, international crime, environmental degradation and infectious diseases, especially HIV/AIDS [1].''

HIV is spread by the intimate exchange of bodily fluids between an infected individual and the recipient. The most important fluids are semen, vaginal secretions, blood, and blood products. HIV exists in two predominant forms, known as HIV-1 and HIV-2. There are significant differences in the amino acid sequences between these two forms of HIV, and in fact HIV-2 differs by more than 55% from HIV-1, as determined by cloning and DNA sequence analysis [4]. The differences between these two forms of HIV continues to have a significant impact in the effectiveness of current drug therapies. In particular, most new therapeutics are designed to inhibit HIV-1, the predominant viral form found in Europe, Asia, much of sub-Saharan Africa, and United States. HIV-2 is the form of the virus most commonly found in western Africa, and is generally a less virulent form of the virus [2].

The HIV virus is capable of rapid replication [3]; however, the viral replication process is prone to frequent polymerization errors that result in the production of viral forms harboring nucleotide mutations and consequently amino acid substitutions. The low-fidelity polymerization process results in the generation of multiple viral subtypes (quasispecies) within an individual. The relative population of these viral subtypes is not static and reflects a natural selection response to pressures induced by various drug therapies and the immune response. The rapid emergence of mutant viral forms under the selective pressure of an antiviral agent increases the difficulty in identifying durable drug therapies and necessitates the use of multiple drugs in order to suppress viral replication.

## IDENTIFICATION OF EFFECTIVE TREATMENTS

The recognition that HIV is a retrovirus, or more precisely a lentivirus, enabled a detailed examination of the replicative process and an identification of enzymes required for viral replication [4]. Three critical enzymes are located within the virion: reverse transcriptase (RT), aspartyl protease, and integrase. RT possesses DNA polymerase and RnaseH activity and is the enzyme responsible for processing viral RNA into proviral DNA [5]. Protease is required for cleavage of *gag* and *gag-pol* precursor proteins into the functional enzymes that are essential for viral replication and the structural proteins required for virus particle assembly. Integrase plays an essential role in the incorporation of proviral DNA into the host cells genome. Detailed knowledge of these critical enzymes enabled the development of reliable biological assays, assays that were needed for drug screening and drug selection.

The realization that HIV was a retrovirus initiated the search for antiviral drugs that would be effective in inhibiting viral replication. This work resulted in the identification of a class of compounds known as nucleoside reverse transcriptase inhibitors (NRTIs) [6]. The NRTIs are substrate decoys for naturally occuring nucleosides, but lack $3'$-hydroxyl groups required for nucleotide polymerization, and thus inhibit the viral RT by intracellular conversion into the active triphosphate form and then binding to the dNTP-binding site of RT. The enzyme-bound NRTI is then incorporated into the growing strand of proviral DNA. Since the NRTI lacks a $3'$-hydroxyl group, the DNA strand is incapable of continued elongation that results in DNA chain termination.

One of the issues that has emerged with the NRTI class of compounds is the long-term, dose-limiting toxicity that results from a complex combination of myelosuppression, bone marrow toxicity, and incorporation into mitochondrial DNA through interaction with cellular DNA polymerases because of a lack of high specificity for HIV-1 RT [7]. Another issue surrounding the NRTIs is the rapid development of resistant strains of virus during the administration of these drugs as monotherapy [8]. This led to the issuance of FDA guidelines requiring drug dosing regimens consisting of multiple NRTIs. There are currently six FDA approved NRTIs on the market: zidovudine (AZT, ZDV), didanosine (ddI), zalcitabine (ddC), stavudine (d4T), lamivudine (3TC) and abacavir (a guanosine analog).

A further advance in HIV therapy was achieved with the development of protease inhibitors (PIs) and the introduction of triple combination therapy consisting of two nucleosides and a protease inhibitor. The inclusion of PIs in drug dosing regimens had a tremendous positive impact on patient longevity: contracting the disease no longer meant certain, relatively rapid death. Issues with the PIs that have limited their effectiveness include problems with their pharmacokinetic, biopharmaceutical or toxicological profiles. For instance, a poor pharmacokinetic profile results in the need to administer large quantities of drug, which in turn drives up the cost of the medication and exacerbates any drug induced side-effects. Furthermore, the pill burden on the patient can become staggering. Using nelfinavir as an example, the adult dosage is 750 mg three times a day (tid): a total of 2.25 grams of drug. Other issues that adversely impact the patients' quality of life with some members of this class of drugs have been the effect of food on gastrointestinal absorption of drug [9] and adverse events [10] such as lipodystrophy and altered lipid metabolism [11]. Using indinavir as an example, the patient is required to take their dose at least 1 hour before a meal or 2 hours after a meal without food but with water. Poor compliance with the complicated dosing regimen can produce blood levels of drug below those needed to inhibit the virus. This results in selective pressure on the virus to evolve mutant viral forms, with the concomitant emergence of protease resistant virus.

Concurrent with the development of the first PIs, another class of compounds was brought to market: the non-nucleoside reverse transcriptase inhibitors (NNRTIs) [12]. Some NNRTIs suffer from a similar liability as found with the PIs: a complicated drug dosing regimen or high pill burden. In particular, the NNRTI nevirapine requires a lead in dosing of two weeks during which time the drug is taken once-a-day (qd), after which the drug is given twice a day (bid). Delavirdine requires doses three times daily. NNRTI toxicities are also problematic: rash is a frequent side effect in patients receiving nevirapine. This adverse reaction can progress to an extremely severe and a potentially fatal condition known as Stevens-Johnson syndrome. In addition, the first generation of NNRTIs suffered from the rapid loss of activity following the emergence of single amino acid mutations in RT.

DISCOVERY AND DEVELOPMENT OF SUSTIVA[TM] (EFAVIRENZ)

After having discovered relatively effective drug treatments for HIV-1 infection, an increasing amount of attention was turned to improving the quality of life for those afflicted with the disease [13]. This could be achieved by reducing the incidence and severity of the side effects caused by the drug regimens, decreasing the pill burden, and simplifying the dosing regimen. The remainder of this chapter describes how drug discovery and development at DuPont Pharmaceuticals was used to achieve a major advance in the ability to increase the quality of life of those suffering from HIV and AIDS.

Discovery of the second generation NNRTIs which were advanced into clinical trials at the DuPont Pharmaceuticals Company (DuPont) is a story which is intimately connected with NNRTI research conducted at Merck & Co. Inc. (Merck). For that reason, a brief historical overview of Merck's contribution to the development of NNRTIs is necessary.

A significant effort at Merck directed toward identifying effective treatments for HIV-1 had been underway for approximately six years at the time of the formation of the DuPont Merck Pharmaceutical Company, a joint venture between DuPont and Merck initiated in 1991. In addition to Merck's pioneering efforts in the development of potent inhibitors of the viral protease, the efforts at Merck led to the identification of a variety of NNRTIs of varying potency and effectiveness, such as the 3-sulfonylindoles (L-737,126 and **1**) [14] and 2-pyridinones (L-697,661 and L-697,639) (*Figure 3.1*) [15,16]. Several 2-pyridinones, including L-697,661, were advanced into phase I clinical trials as monotherapy and were subsequently abandoned because of the rapid development of resistant strains of HIV [16,17]. The results from this study indicated that when L-697,661 was used in combination with the NRTI zidovudine (also

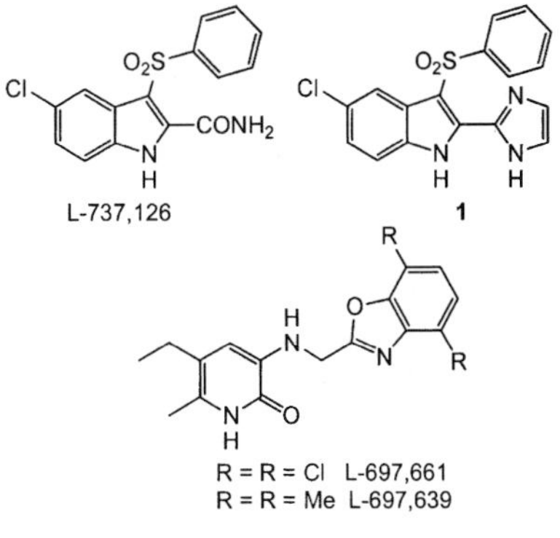

L-737,126

**1**

R = R = Cl  L-697,661
R = R = Me  L-697,639

*Figure 3.1.*

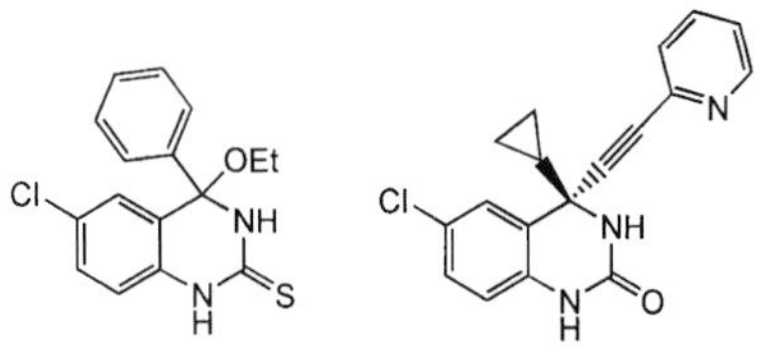

L-608,788          L-738,372

*Figure 3.2.*

known as AZT or ZDV), the development of viral strains highly resistant to the 2-pyridinone could be avoided. This observation led to the initiation of a phase II clinical trial wherein L-697,661 was co-administered with zidovudine [18]. The results from this study indicated that it was possible to delay the development of strains of virus resistant to the pyridinone by approximately 10 weeks [19]. The clinical significance of this result was determined to be questionable, and this compound was not developed further. L-697,639, another 2-pyridinone, was advanced into phase I clinical trials and development was also subsequently discontinued [20].

Screening the compound repository at Merck for other novel compounds which possessed anti-HIV RT activity resulted in the identification of the unstable quinazolin-2(1*H*)-thione hemiacetal L-608,788 [21]. Extensive SAR studies on the quinazolinones led to the identification of the 2-pyridylacetylene-containing quinazolinone L-738,372 as a potent NNRTI and this compound was selected for development [22–24].

As part of Merck's continuing research effort at identifying new NNRTIs, the benzoxazinone ring system was evaluated. This effort eventually led to the identification of L-743,726 [25]. Merck out-licensed the development rights of L-743,726 to the DuPont Merck Pharmaceutical Company during the formation of the joint venture. L-743,726 came to be known as DMP-266 and later as

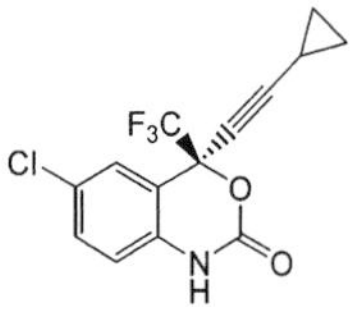

L-743,726
DMP-266
efavirenz

*Figure 3.3.*

efavirenz. DuPont sells efavirenz under the trademark SUSTIVA$^{TM}$ and Merck sells efavirenz under the trademark STOCRIN$^{TM}$.

Efavirenz is a potent, selective inhibitor with an IC$_{90}$ of $\sim 2\,nM$ toward wild-type virus and many single mutant forms of HIV-1 RT. Efavirenz was the first NNRTI to be listed by the FDA as a preferred first-line therapy since efavirenz was shown to be highly efficacious when used with two NRTIs in a protease-sparing regimen [26]. Efavirenz is also administered along with two NRTIs in protease inhibitor-containing drug regimens. The protease-sparing regimen results in a substantially decreased pill burden for the patient, which in turn results in a simplification of the dosing schedule and an increase in patient compliance. The decrease in the pill burden is dramatic: three 200 mg efavirenz tablets once-daily and one Combivir$^{TM}$ (AZT/3TC combination) tablet twice-daily for a total of five pills. The absence of a food effect with efavirenz or with preferred NRTIs further simplifies the dosing schedule. The use of a protease-sparing regimen has another benefit which is that protease inhibitors can theoretically be saved for when/if the patient develops resistance to one of the components of the efavirenz/NRTI therapy.

The majority of patients receiving efavirenz-containing regimens have shown sustained antiviral responses. However, greater than 90% of those patients whose viral loads have rebounded after an initial response to drug contain the asparagine to lysine point mutation at position 103 (K103N mutation) [27]. Additional double mutant forms of virus emerge more slowly following the development of the K103N mutation [28]. In particular, within four months after the initial viral load rebound, the double mutations K103N-V108I or K103N-P225H are observed in a large number of samples [27]. These observations indicated that there was a need to identify NNRTIs which would be capable of suppressing the viral replication of singly and doubly mutated HIV-1 RT viral forms containing the K103N mutation when combined with other highly active antiretroviral therapies (HAART). Such an agent could be the cornerstone of therapeutic regimens for individuals already experienced with and resistant to the NNRTI class. It was also desirable to discover drugs that would retain the ease of administration and safety profile of efavirenz: i.e., once-daily dosing, no food effect and minimal adverse effects.

Another of the issues related to the administration of efavirenz was the observation that the P450 liver isozyme CYP3A4 was upregulated. This particular isozyme is responsible for the metabolism of members of the protease inhibitor class. The end result of the upregulation of CYP3A4 is that the dosage of protease inhibitors may need to be increased to compensate for more rapid clearance with increased CYP3A4 activity. Thus, identification of a second generation NNRTI that did not induce CYP3A4 was also desirable. It is worth noting that decreased exposure to a PI upon administration of an NNRTI is not unique to efavirenz: nevirapine decreases saquinavir and indinavir exposure levels by 30% [29].

## STATUS OF NNRTI RESEARCH – 1995

The initial goals at DuPont Merck were to understand the SAR regarding the upregulation of CYP3A4 using the benzoxazinone core structure found in efavirenz and to identify compounds that showed an improved resistance profile, particularly against the K103N single mutation. It was hoped that both objectives could be achieved through the judicious choice of appropriate groups on either the aromatic ring or on the alkyne, or perhaps replacement of the alkyne with other groups.

### BENZOXAZINONE SAR

A portion of the SAR work surrounding the benzoxazinone core is summarized in *Tables 3.1* through *3.3* (see *Figure 3.4* for generic structural representations). Initially, the effect of manipulating the functional groups on

Table 3.1   BENZOXAZINONE SAR: EFFECT OF VARYING AROMATIC SUBSTITUTION

| | | | | | $IC_{50}(nM)$ | Wild-Type | K103N |
|---|---|---|---|---|---|---|---|
| | | X | | | | | |
| Compound | 5 | 6 | 7 | 8 | [31a] | $IC_{90}(nM)$ [31b] | $IC_{90}(nM)$ |
| **Efavirenz** | H | Cl | H | H | 48 | 2.0 | $64 \pm 24$ |
| **2** | H | H | H | H | 478 | 10 | 1320 |
| **3** | H | F | H | H | 190 | 7.4 | 535 |
| **4** | H | i-Pr | H | H | 1958 | 28 | $ND^a$ |
| **5** | H | N(Me)$_2$ | H | H | 816 | 8.3 | 956 |
| **6** | H | OCF$_3$ | H | H | 1249 | 19 | 1010 |
| **7** | F | F | H | H | 84 | 3.2 | 72.5 |
| **8** | F | H | H | F | 796 | 18.0 | $ND^a$ |
| **9** | F | F | H | F | 800 | 14 | $ND^a$ |
| **10** | F | F | F | H | 442 | 20 | $ND^a$ |
| **11** | H | F | F | F | >2000 | 418 | $ND^a$ |
| **12** | H | Cl | H | OMe | $ND^a$ | 122 | $ND^a$ |
| **13** | H | Cl | H | Cl | >2000 | 29 | $ND^a$ |
| **14** | H | OMe | H | H | 131 | 2 | 167 |
| **15** | H | Cl | H | F | $ND^a$ | 7.2 | 777 |
| **16** | H | Ph | H | H | >2000 | 249 | $ND^a$ |
| **17** | H | Me | H | H | 133 | 7.1 | $ND^a$ |
| **18** | H | $-CH=CH-CH=CH-$ | | H | 1909 | 27 | $ND^a$ |

$^a$ND = Not Determined.

Table 3.2.  BENZOXAZINONE SAR: EFFECT OF VARYING AROMATIC AND ALKYNYL
SUBSTITUTION

$X$

| Compound | 5 | 6 | R | Enzyme $IC_{50}$ (nM) [31a] | Wild-Type $IC_{90}$ (nM) [31b] |
|----------|---|---|---|------|------|
| Efavirenz | H | Cl | cyclopropyl | 48 | 2.0 |
| 19 | F | H | cyclopropyl | 78 | 4.3 |
| 20 | F | H | Ethyl | 127 | 4.2 |
| 21 | F | H | n-propyl | 156 | 5.6 |
| 22 | F | H | isopropyl | 102 | 6.6 |
| 23 | H | NO$_2$ | cyclopropyl | 209 | 0.8 |
| 24 | H | NO$_2$ | ethyl | 276 | 2.2 |
| 25 | H | NO$_2$ | n-propyl | 304 | 4.6 |
| 26 | H | NO$_2$ | i-propyl | 199 | 3.4 |
| 27 | H | NH$_2$ | cyclopropyl | 802 | 21 |
| 28 | H | NH$_2$ | ethyl | 1894 | 46 |
| 29 | H | NH$_2$ | n-propyl | 1506 | 34 |
| 30 | H | NH$_2$ | i-propyl | 896 | 27 |
| 31 | H | N(H)Me | cyclopropyl | 608 | 9.0 |
| 32 | H | N(H)Me | i-propyl | 473 | 10 |
| 33 | H | N(H)Ac | cyclopropyl | >2000 | 296 |
| 34 | H | N(H)Ac | i-propyl | >2000 | 500 |

the aromatic ring was evaluated and these results are shown in *Table 3.1*
[30,31]. These studies revealed that the 5,6-difluoro derivative **7** possessed
activity toward wild-type virus similar to that of efavirenz [32]. The only other
compound which possessed activity similar to that of efavirenz was the 6-
methoxy derivative **14**.

The effect of varying the alkyne and the nature of the aromatic substitution in
benzoxazinones was evaluated further and the data presented in *Table 3.2* [33].
The incorporation of a nitro group into the 6-position resulted in compound **23**
which possessed sub-nanomolar activity in the antiviral assay and had an
$IC_{90} = 59$ nM against the K103N RT mutant, while efavirenz had K103N
$IC_{90} = 64$ nM. The cyclopropyl and isopropyl alkynes were essentially equipotent for all aromatic substitutions examined. In general, electron withdrawing
groups on the aromatic ring resulted in more active compounds and minimal
effects on the biological activity were observed by varying the nature of small
alkyne groups.

Next, the incorporation of heteroaryl alkynes into benzoxazinones was
explored using several different halogen substitutions on the aromatic ring
(*Table 3.3*) [34,36]. 3-Pyridyl alkyne substituted benzoxazinones were found to
be potent NNRTIs, as evidenced by the activity of **36**, **43** and **49**: wild-type
$IC_{90}$s = 4, 3 and 2 nM, respectively. In fact, a variety of small heterocycles

Table 3.3.  BENZOXAZINONE SAR: INCORPORATION OF HETERARYL ALKYNES

| | X | | | Wild-Type | K103N | L100I |
|---|---|---|---|---|---|---|
| Compound | 5 | 6 | R | $IC_{90}$ (nM) [31b] | $IC_{90}$ (nM) | $IC_{90}$ (nM) |
| **Efavirenz** | H | Cl | cyclopropyl | 2.0 | 64 | $ND^a$ |
| 35 | H | Cl | 2-Pyridyl | 5.4 | 1106 | $ND^a$ |
| 36 | H | Cl | 3-Pyridyl | 4.0 | 145 | $ND^a$ |
| 37 | H | Cl | 4-Pyridyl | 102 | $ND^a$ | $ND^a$ |
| 38 | H | Cl | 2-Furanyl | 3.8 | 152 | 167 |
| 39 | H | Cl | 3-Furanyl | 3.8 | 322 | 170 |
| 40 | H | Cl | 3-Thienyl | 4.5 | 106 | 115 |
| 41 | H | Cl | 5-Thiazolyl | 6.7 | $ND^a$ | $ND^a$ |
| 42 | H | F | 2-Pyridyl | 12 | $ND^a$ | $ND^a$ |
| 43 | H | F | 3-Pyridyl | 2.6 | 329 | $ND^a$ |
| 44 | H | F | 2-Furanyl | 2.6 | $ND^a$ | $ND^a$ |
| 45 | H | F | 3-Furanyl | 2.5 | 369 | 256 |
| 46 | H | F | 2-Thienyl | 2.9 | $ND^a$ | $ND^a$ |
| 47 | H | F | 3-Thienyl | 2.6 | 193 | 211 |
| 48 | F | F | 2-Pyridyl | 6.8 | $ND^a$ | $ND^a$ |
| 49 | F | F | 3-Pyridyl | 2.2 | 59 | $ND^a$ |
| 50 | F | F | 2-Furanyl | 3.8 | $ND^a$ | $ND^a$ |
| 51 | F | F | 3-Furanyl | 3.2 | 280 | 179 |
| 52 | F | F | 2-Thienyl | 2.2 | 156 | $ND^a$ |
| 53 | F | F | 3-Thienyl | 2.3 | 139 | 106 |

$^a$ND = Not Determined.

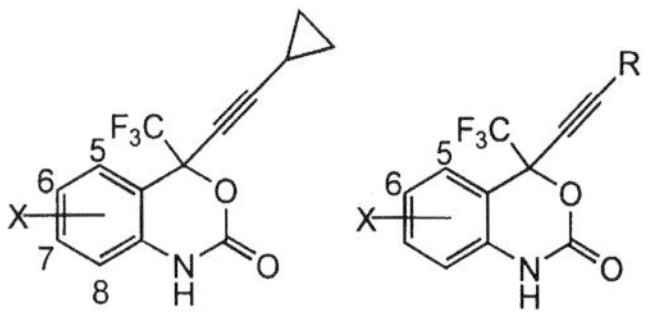

Figure 3.4.

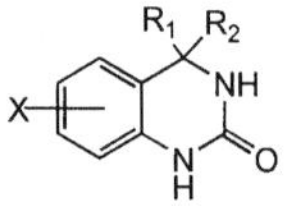

Figure 3.5.

were also very potent inhibitors of wild-type HIV-1 RT. Interestingly, the 3-pyridyl acetylene **49** exhibited good activity against the problematic K103N single mutation as evidenced by its 59 nM $IC_{90}$.

## TRIFLUOROMETHYL-CONTAINING QUINAZOLIN-2(1*H*)-ONES

Concurrent with the exploration of the SAR of the benzoxazinone ring system as illustrated in *Tables 3.1* through *3.3*, an effort was made to identify other heterocycles that would function as NNRTIs and satisfy the objectives of increased potency against mutant virus forms and decreased CYP3A4 induction. As has been previously discussed, quinazolin-2(1*H*)-ones had already been identified by Merck as potent NNRTIs, with the Achilles heel being the rapid emergence of resistant virus. However, the discovery of efavirenz had revealed that the trifluoromethyl group played a critical role in imparting beneficial activity toward mutant forms of HIV-1 RT. Furthermore, the beneficial impact of the cyclopropyl acetylene group in efavirenz on the resistance profile was also becoming more evident: small alkyl acetylenes were needed for a good resistance profile, with the possible exception to this being the 3-pyridyl acetylene derivatives. The question arose as to whether similar modifications (incorporation of a trifluoromethyl group and a cyclopropyl acetylene) into a quinazolin-2(1*H*)-one would impart an improvement in the resistance profile.

### PREPARATION OF QUINAZOLINONES – BACKGROUND

Merck's route to the quinazolinone ring system is exemplified through the preparation of their clinical candidate L-738,372. The first step involved adding a Grignard reagent to 2-amino-5-chlorobenzonitrile **(54)** and trapping the *in situ* generated imine anion with dimethyl carbonate (*Figure 3.6*) [21a]. The *N*-1 of the resultant ketimine **55** was protected with a *p*-methoxybenzyl (PMB) group, ketimine **56** was then precomplexed with magnesium triflate and the lithiated 2-pyridylacetylide was added to afford the 4,4-disubstituted quinazolinone **57**. It was necessary to precomplex ketimine **56** with a Lewis acid in order to avoid reduction of the ketimine to the saturated system, a reaction which proved problematic at DuPont Pharmaceuticals during the addition of Grignard reagents to a similarly functionalized trifluoromethyl-substituted ketimine (*vida supra*). The PMB group was subsequently removed with trifluoroacetic acid to afford the desired product **58**. Alternatively, *N*-3 of **57** could be alkylated using iodomethane in DMF containing sodium hydride followed by PMB removal to deliver 4,4-disubstituted, *N*-3 alkyl quinazolinone **59**.

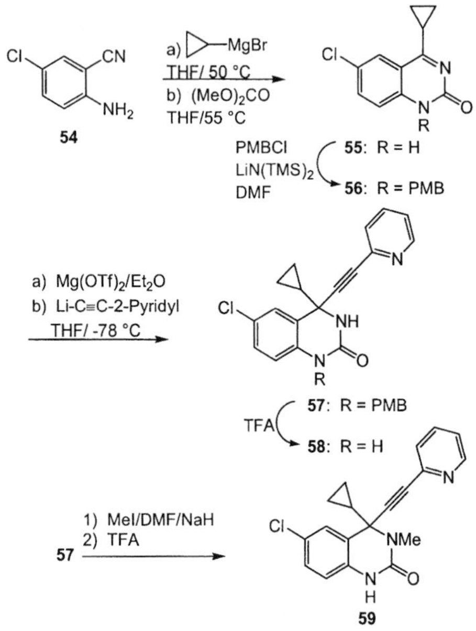

Figure 3.6.

## PREPARATION OF TRIFLUOROMETHYL-CONTAINING QUINAZOLINONES

The route shown in *Figure 3.6* could be modified to produce the various tri-fluoromethyl-containing quinazolinones. This required preparing appropriately substituted *o*-amino-trifluoromethylketones. Fortunately, it was possible to obtain large quantities of the 1-(2-amino-5-chloro)-2,2,2-trifluoroethanone (60) since it is a trifluoromethyl ketone used in the preparation of efavirenz (*Figure 3.7*). Therefore, initial synthetic efforts at preparing 4-trifluoromethyl-substituted quinazolinones utilized ketone 60.

The first route explored consisted of treating ketone 60 with trimethylsily-lisocyanate in tetrahydrofuran (THF) with catalytic dimethylaminopyridine (DMAP) followed by a solution of tetrabutylammonium flouride in THF to deliver aminol 61 (*Figure 3.7*) [35]. It was later found that the preparation of 61 proceeded in much higher yields, more reproducibly and could be isolated in greater purity by performing the same transformation using potassium cyanate in an acetic acid/water mixture. Heating 61 at reflux in toluene containing 4 Å molecular sieves dehydrated the aminol and afforded ketimine 62.

Treating 62 with lithium bistrimethylsilyamide and *p*-methoxybenzyl chloride was expected to afford the desired *N*-1 protected derivative 63

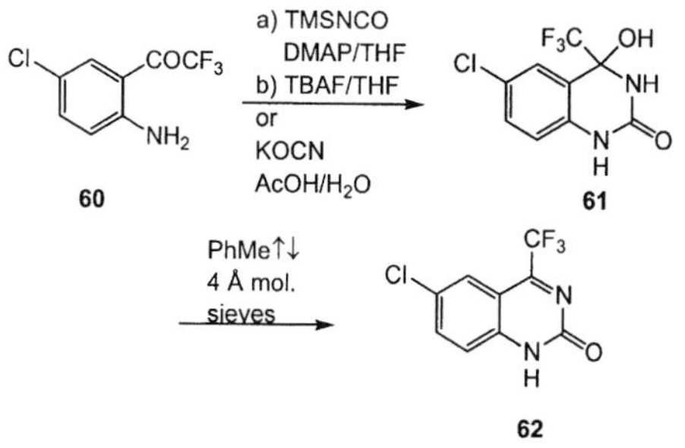

Figure 3.7.

(*Figure 3.8*). However, the conditions afforded a mixture of the desired material **63**, as the minor component, along with another material presumed to be the α-chloro compound **64**. The electron withdrawing properties of the trifluoromethyl group activated the imine and prevented the isolation of the desired material. Initially, attempts were made to use the inseparable mixture of **63** and **64** since it could be rationalized that upon treatment with an excess of lithiated acetylide, **64** could be converted into **63** upon deprotonation of the hydrogen at *N*-3. In the event, treating **63** and **64** with an excess of cyclopropyl acetylide in THF returned unreacted **64** and minor amounts of the desired adduct **65**. The amount of **65** obtained was approximately equivalent to the amount of **63** present in the mixture of **63** and **64**. Therefore, **64** was not converted into **63** under these reaction conditions.

The ability of the lithiated acetylide to add to **63** combined with the observation that the imine carbon bearing the trifluoromethyl group preferred

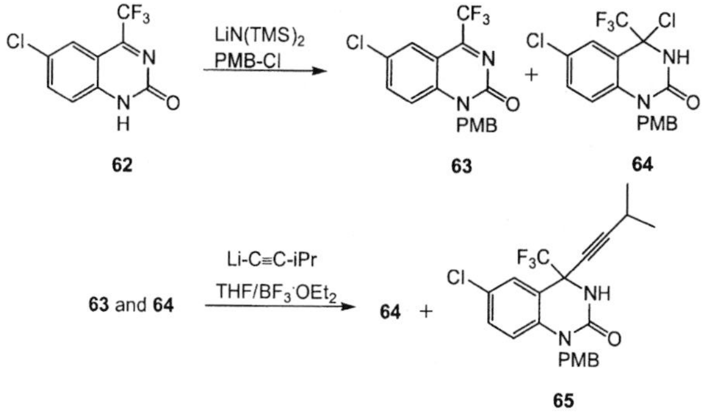

Figure 3.8.

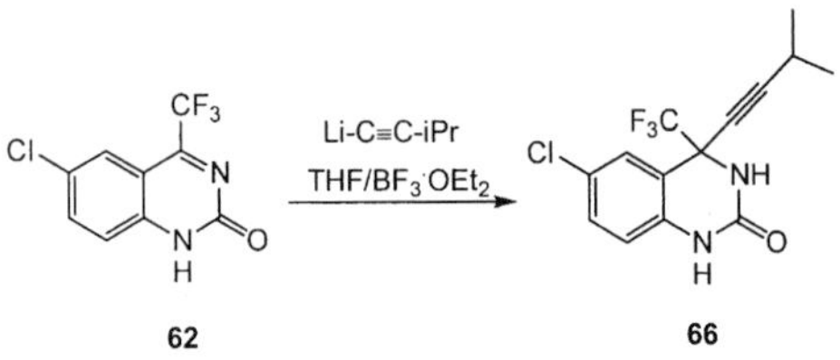

*Figure 3.9.*

being sp3 hybridized, as in **64**, were the observations which resulted in a satisfactory solution. That solution entailed treating ketimine **62** with lithiated acetylides, first exemplified by 3-methyl-1-butynyl acetylide, in the presence of 0.5 equivalents of boron trifluoride diethyl etherate ($BF_3 \cdot OEt_2$) in THF (*Figure 3.9*). The desired adduct **66** was obtained in high yield without the use of any protecting groups, and in only three steps from a material available in metric ton quantities. It would latter be demonstrated in *Figure 3.12* that various lithiocarbanions, not just lithiated alkynes, could be successfully added to trifluoromethyl-containing ketimines (as demonstrated by compounds **119**, **121**, **123**, **125** and **127** in *Table 3.6*).

With a route to the desired compounds identified, a variety of substituted aromatic compounds were prepared. The synthesis of some of the requisite starting materials had already been achieved during the SAR work on the benzoxazinones. For instance, the preparation of 3-halo anilino ketones **80** and

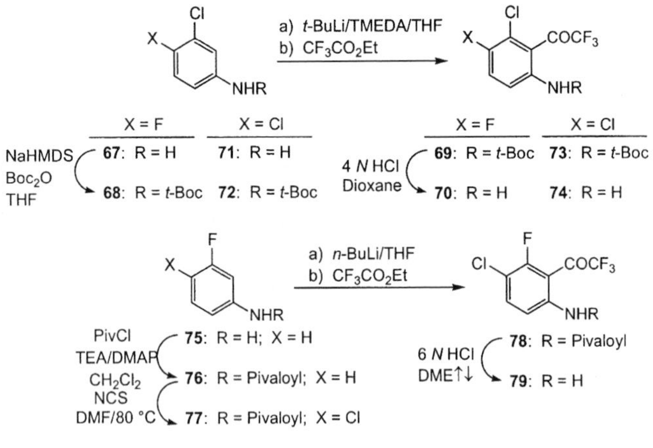

*Figure 3.10.*

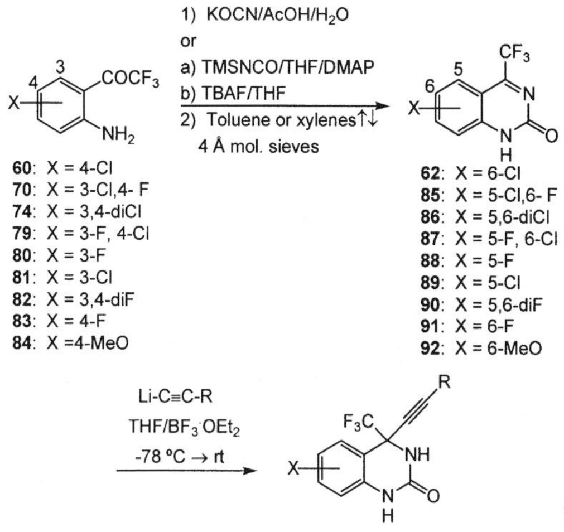

1) KOCN/AcOH/H₂O
or
a) TMSNCO/THF/DMAP
b) TBAF/THF
2) Toluene or xylenes↑↓
4 Å mol. sieves

60: X = 4-Cl
70: X = 3-Cl,4- F
74: X = 3,4-diCl
79: X = 3-F, 4-Cl
80: X = 3-F
81: X = 3-Cl
82: X = 3,4-diF
83: X = 4-F
84: X =4-MeO

62: X = 6-Cl
85: X = 5-Cl,6- F
86: X = 5,6-diCl
87: X = 5-F, 6-Cl
88: X = 5-F
89: X = 5-Cl
90: X = 5,6-diF
91: X = 6-F
92: X = 6-MeO

Li-C≡C-R
THF/BF₃ OEt₂
-78 °C → rt

*Figure 3.11.*

**81**, 3,4-difluoro, 4-fluoro, and 4-methoxy anilino ketones **82**, **83** and **84**, respectively, had already been accomplished (*Figure 3.11*) [30, 33]. The preparation of the dihalogenated benzoxazinones indicated that these compounds possessed good biological activity and, in some cases, had lower protein binding compared to the 6-chloroderivatives. These observations were the impetus behind preparing dihalogen-substituted quinazolinones. The preparation of the requisite *o*-amino-trifluoromethyl ketone starting materials that had not previously been prepared is shown in *Figure 3.10*. 3-Chloro-4-fluoroaniline (**67**) was protected with a *t*-Boc group, and **68** underwent a directed ortho-metallation (DOM) followed by quenching of the anion with ethyl trifluoroacetate to deliver the desired ketone **69**. Removal of the *t*-Boc protecting group afforded the desired material, ketone **70**. Starting with 3,4-dichloroaniline (**71**), a similar approach was followed to prepare the 3,4-dichloro derivative **74**. The synthetic route to 3-fluoro, 4-chloroanilino ketone **79** began by first protecting 3-fluoroaniline (**75**) with a pivaloyl group, chlorinating **76** with *N*-chlorosuccinimide upon brief heating in DMF to afford **77**, performing a DOM using *n*-butyllithium and quenching the anion with ethyltrifluoroacetate gave **78**. Removal of the pivaloyl group from **78** completed the preparation of **79**.

Ketones **60**, **70**, **74**, **79** and **80–84** [30,33] were transformed in two steps into ketimines **62** and **85–92**. In *Figure 3.11* is a generic representation of the chemistry utilized to prepare 4-trifluoromethyl, 4-alkyne-substituted quinazolinones. The reactions afforded product in a modest yield, with the highest yields generally occurring with the 6-chloro ketimine **62**. All attempts at preparing 3-pyridyl derivatives via this route failed. However, work performed latter in the project, and presented in *Figure 3.10*, revealed a synthetic route which was used to access the 3-pyridyl quinazolinone **189**. The 5,6-difluoro, 3-pyridylquinazolinone **189** had modest biological activity (*Table 3.11*).

The potency of the alkynyl-substituted quinazolinones in an HIV-1 RT *in vitro* enzyme assay ($IC_{50}$ data) [3la] and against the wild-type RF strain of HIV-1 ($IC_{90}$ data) [3lb] are shown in *Table 3.4*, with efavirenz included for comparison. Many drugs bind to plasma proteins. Because only unbound drug is freely diffusable, the effect of this plasma protein binding is to decrease the

Table 3.4.  ANTIVIRAL POTENCY OF TRIFLUOROMETHYL-CONTAINING QUINAZOLINONES

| Compound | X | R | Enzyme $IC_{50}$ (nM) [31a] | $IC_{90}$ (nM) Antiviral Activity [31b] | PB Adj. Wild Type | PB Fold Shift |
|---|---|---|---|---|---|---|
| **93** | 5,6-diF | Ethyl | $74 \pm 27$ | 1.5 | 10 | 7 |
| **94** | 5-F | Cyclopropyl | $62 \pm 13$ | 1.4 | 14 | 10 |
| **95** | 5,Cl,6-F | *i*-Propyl | $78 \pm 25$ | 3.0 | 15 | 5 |
| **96** | 5-Cl | Cyclopropyl | $72 \pm 15$ | 2.5 | 18 | 7 |
| **97** | 5,6-diF | Cyclopropyl | $74 \pm 35$ | 2.1 | 19 | 9 |
| **98** | 5,6-diF | *i*-Propyl | $91 \pm 13$ | $2.1 \pm 1.4$ | 21 | 10 |
| **99** | 6-F | Cyclopropyl | $50 \pm 4$ | 2.0 | 24 | 12 |
| **100** | 5,6-diF | 2-Pyridyl | $68 \pm 17$ | 2.0 | 24 | 12 |
| **101** | 6-F | Ethyl | $54 \pm 9$ | 2.5 | 25 | 10 |
| **102** | 5,Cl,6-F | Cyclopropyl | $59 \pm 12$ | 2.7 | 27 | 10 |
| **Efavirenz** | | | $47 \pm 25$ | $1.7 \pm 0.5$ | 28 | 16.5 |
| **103** | 6-MeO | Cyclopropyl | $124 \pm 90$ | 2.9 | 29 | 10 |
| **104** | 6-F | 2-Pyridyl | $126 \pm 30$ | 5 | 33 | 7 |
| **105** | 5-F,6-Cl | Cyclopropyl | $102 \pm 67$ | 4.8 | 40 | 8.4 |
| **106** | 5-Cl,6-F | 2-Pyridyl | $80 \pm 15$ | 2.3 | 41 | 18 |
| **107** | 6-Cl | Cyclopropyl | $111 \pm 34$ | $2.7 \pm 0.6$ | 41 | 15 |
| **108** | 6-MeO | *i*-Propyl | $401 \pm 182$ | 3.8 | 42 | 11 |
| **109** | 6-MeO | Phenyl | $219 \pm 34$ | 3.2 | 42 | 13 |
| **110** | 5,6-diF | Phenyl | $181 \pm 83$ | 6.2 | 43 | 7 |
| **111** | 6-F | Phenyl | $143 \pm 30$ | 6.6 | 66 | 10 |
| **112** | 6-Cl | 2-Pyridyl | $129 \pm 36$ | 3.4 | 79 | 23 |
| **113** | 6-Cl | Ethyl | $110 \pm 61$ | 3.3 | 83 | 25 |
| **114** | 6-Cl | Phenyl | $277 \pm 94$ | 7.1 | 86 | 12 |
| **115** | 6-F | *i*-Propyl | $39 \pm 8$ | 2.6 | 86 | 33 |
| **116** | 5,6-diCl | Cyclopropyl | $166 \pm 38$ | 8.0 | 88 | 11 |
| **117** | 6-Cl | *i*-Propyl | $281 \pm 105$ | $3.0 \pm 0.2$ | 90 | 30 |
| **118** | 6-MeO | 2-Pyridyl | $237 \pm 99$ | 8.1 | 138 | 17 |

drug available to enter cells and bind to the intracellular target. We therefore developed an assay that enabled the rapid estimation of protein binding by determining the influence of added serum proteins on the antiviral potency in cell culture. The serum proteins examined were human serum albumin (HSA) and α-acid glycoprotein (AAG) at concentrations found in human serum (45 mg/mL HSA and 1 mg/mL AAG). The antiviral potency was then determined by measurement of viral RNA in standard tissue culture medium and in tissue culture medium to which HSA and AAG had been added. The ratio of the measured 90% inhibitory concentrations was then expressed as a fold-increase in measured $IC_{90}$ (i.e., the PB fold shift).

Most of the quinazolinones in *Table 3.4* had anti-viral ($IC_{90}$) potency similar to efavirenz. However, when the estimated amount of protein binding was taken into account, significant differences between efavirenz and the quinazolinones became apparent [36]. A halogen substituent in the 5-position, either in the presence or absence of a halogen substituent in the 6-position, conferred beneficial activity: eight of the top ten compounds possessing protein binding adjusted wild-type $IC_{90}$ values less than efavirenz are either 5-monohalogen or 5,6-dihalogenated quinazolinones. Compounds with a phenyl-substituted alkyne were less potent, while some compounds possessing a 2-pyridyl acetylene group had potency similar to efavirenz (compounds **100** and **104**). The 2-pyridyl-containing quinazolinones **100** and **104** were less active, however, than their corresponding cyclopropyl alkynyl (**97** and **99**, respectively) and butyn-1-yl (**93** and **101**, respectively) analogues.

The modest improvement in the protein binding adjusted wild-type activity observed for some of the quinazolinones over efavirenz is attributed to a decrease in the protein binding since the antiviral activity is essentially the same for efavirenz as for the most active quinazolinones. The improvement of the quinazolinones over the benzoxazinones became even more evident when we examined the antiviral efficacy of these compounds against the K103N and L100I HIV-1 RT mutant variants. The K103N mutant is clinically significant since it is the most prevalent mutation observed *in vivo* in patients who have failed efavirenz-containing therapies [37]. This particular mutation is frequently observed as a single mutation or in combination with other mutations in nevirapine and delavirdine treatment failures [27,28]. Another mutation which has been frequently observed during *in vitro* selection experiments with efavirenz is L100I [31b]. The data in *Table 3.5* are ranked according to the protein binding adjusted antiviral potency toward the K103N HIV-1 RT mutant. Eighteen compounds were more potent than efavirenz against the K103N mutant as the racemates; the most potent compound, **95**, was 14-times more potent against K103N. This improvement in protein binding-adjusted potency results from increased potency and smaller protein binding shift. The most active compounds all possessed a 5,6-dihalogen substitution and they had small

Table 3.5.  ANTIVIRAL POTENCY OF QUINAZOLINONES RANKED BY PROTEIN
BINDING ADJUSTED ACTIVITY AGAINST K103N MUTATION

| | | | $IC_{90}$ (nM) | | |
|---|---|---|---|---|---|
| Compound | X | R | Antiviral Activity K103N | Antiviral Activity L100I | PB Adj. K103N |
| 95 | 5-Cl, 6-F | i-Propyl | 15 | 13 | 74 |
| 93 | 5,6-diF | Ethyl | 14 | 18 | 93 |
| 97 | 5,6-diF | Cyclopropyl | 13 | 12 | 119 |
| 98 | 5,6-diF | i-Propyl | 14 | 10 | 139 |
| 105 | 5-F, 6-Cl | Cyclopropyl | 18 | ND[a] | 151 |
| 102 | 5-Cl, 6-F | Cyclopropyl | 18 | 16 | 178 |
| 116 | 5,6-diCl | Cyclopropyl | 18 | ND[a] | 196 |
| 107 | 6-Cl | Cyclopropyl | 22 | 18 | 336 |
| 103 | 6-MeO | Cyclopropyl | 40 | 46 | 396 |
| 96 | 5-Cl | Cyclopropyl | 63 | 70 | 441 |
| 99 | 6-F | Cyclopropyl | 48 | 29 | 566 |
| 108 | 6-MeO | i-Propyl | 56 | 28 | 599 |
| 117 | 6-Cl | i-Propyl | 22 | 28 | 653 |
| 101 | 6-F | Ethyl | 71 | 74 | 710 |
| 113 | 6-Cl | Ethyl | 26 | ND[a] | 826 |
| 115 | 6-F | i-Propyl | 27 | 17 | 891 |
| 94 | 5-F | Cyclopropyl | 89 | 108 | 917 |
| Efavirenz | | | $64 \pm 27$ | $77 \pm 26$ | 1056 |
| 106 | 5-Cl, 6-F | 2-Pyridyl | 73 | 44 | 1307 |
| 100 | 5,6-diF | 2-Pyridyl | 109 | 37 | 1308 |
| 110 | 5,6-diF | Phenyl | 191 | 256 | 1337 |
| 114 | 6-Cl | Phenyl | 250 | 365 | 3000 |
| 104 | 6-F | 2-Pyridyl | 483 | 255 | 3140 |
| 111 | 6-F | Phenyl | 322 | 677 | 3220 |
| 109 | 6-MeO | Phenyl | 283 | 462 | 3594 |
| 112 | 6-Cl | 2-Pyridyl | 160 | 64 | 3728 |
| 118 | 6-MeO | 2-Pyridyl | 338 | 98 | 5881 |

[a]ND = Not Determined.

alkyl groups on the alkyne.    The effect upon activity by enhancing the rotational mobility of the alkynyl side chain was explored by synthesizing compounds that lacked the alkynyl-group. These compounds were prepared either by catalytic hydrogenation of the corresponding alkyne or by addition of an alkyllithium to the appropriate ketimine (*Figure 3.12*).

The quinazolinones with increased freedom of rotation possessed good activity against wild-type virus (*Table 3.6*). In fact, the single enantiomers of the 6-fluoro-derivatized materials having the butyl and 3-methyl-1-butynyl groups, compounds **119** and **120**, respectively, would be expected to have protein binding adjusted IC90's less than efavirenz. The analogous derivatives

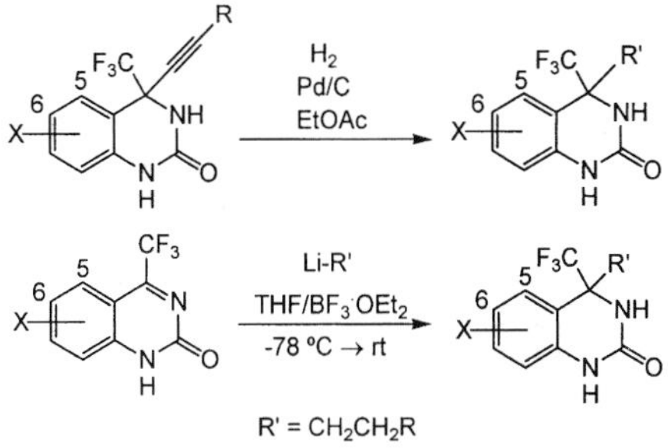

*Figure 3.12.*

possessing the 5,6-difluoroaromatic substitution, **121** and **122**, were only marginally less active. Activity dropped off significantly when large groups were appended to the terminus of the alkyl side chain, as was observed with **124** and **126**. The 2-butyn-1-yl side chain was moderately well accommodated, although it was not as potent as efavirenz. An interesting observation was that some of the alkyl quinazolinones appeared to possess lower protein binding shifts (PB shifts) when compared to the corresponding alkynyl derivatives. For instance, **120** and **115** had PB shifts of 4.2 and 33, respectively, and **122** exhibited a marginally improved PB shift over **98**: 5.5 and 10, respectively.

The activity of these compounds against the K103N mutant is given in *Table 3.7*. Quinazolinone **122** was slightly less potent than the corresponding alkynyl derivative **98** in the K103N antiviral assay, 34 nM and 14 nM, respectively, but

Table 3.6. ANTIVIRAL POTENCY OF ALKYL SUBSTITUTED QUINAZOLINONES

| | | | $IC_{90}$ (nM) | | | |
|---|---|---|---|---|---|---|
| Compound | X | $R'$ | Enzyme $IC_{50}$ (nM) [31a] | Antiviral Activity [31b] | PB Adj. Wild Type | PB Fold Shift |
| **119** | 6-F | $CH_2CH_2CH_2CH_3$ | $93 \pm 36$ | 5.9 | 21 | 3.5 |
| **120** | 6-F | $CH_2CH_2CH(CH_3)_2$ | $131 \pm 24$ | 5.6 | 24 | 4.2 |
| **Efavirenz** | | | $47 \pm 25$ | $1.7 \pm 0.5$ | 28 | 16.5 |
| **121** | 5,6-diF | $CH_2CH_2CH_2CH_3$ | $76 \pm 6$ | 6.5 | 31 | 4.8 |
| **122** | 5,6-diF | $CH_2CH_2CH(CH_3)_2$ | $223 \pm 40$ | 8.4 | 46 | 5.5 |
| **123** | 6-F | $CH_2C \equiv CCH_3$ | $457 \pm 52$ | 15 | 53 | 3.5 |
| **124** | 6-F | $CH_2CH_2$-(2-Pyridyl) | $1532 \pm 177$ | 23 | 168 | 7.3 |
| **125** | 6-Cl | $CH_2CH_2cPr$ | $154 \pm 51$ | 9.7 | $ND^a$ | |
| **126** | 6-F | $CH_2CH_2Ph$ | 2180 | 47 | ND | |
| **127** | 5,6-diF | $CH_2CH_2cPr$ | $135 \pm 23$ | 11.2 | ND | |

$^a$ND = Not Determined.

Table 3.7. ANTIVIRAL POTENCY AGAINST MUTANT VIRAL FORMS

| | | | $IC_{90}$ (nM) | | |
|---|---|---|---|---|---|
| Compound | X | R | Antiviral Activity K103N | Antiviral Activity L100I | PB Adj. K103N |
| 122 | 5,6-diF | $CH_2CH_2CH(CH_3)_2$ | 34 | 9 | 187 |
| 120 | 6-F | $CH_2CH_2CH(CH_3)_2$ | 85 | 26 | 357 |
| 121 | 5,6-diF | $CH_2CH_2CH_2CH_3$ | 78 | 23 | 374 |
| 119 | 6-F | $CH_2CH_2CH_2CH_3$ | 172 | 55 | 602 |
| Efavirenz | | | $64 \pm 27$ | $77 \pm 26$ | 1056 |
| 123 | 6-F | $CH_2C \equiv CCH_3$ | 1852 | 1363 | 6482 |
| 124 | 6-F | $CH_2CH_2$-(2-Pyridyl) | $ND^a$ | $ND^a$ | $ND^a$ |
| 125 | 6-Cl | $CH_2CH_2cPr$ | 377 | $ND^a$ | $ND^a$ |
| 126 | 6-F | $CH_2CH_2Ph$ | $ND^a$ | $ND^a$ | $ND^a$ |
| 127 | 5,6-diF | $CH_2CH_2cPr$ | $ND^a$ | $ND^a$ | $ND^a$ |

$^a$ND = Not Determined.

was less tightly protein bound as evidenced by a lower protein binding shift value. Therefore, **122** was about as active against the K103N mutant in terms of its protein binding adjusted value as **98**: 187 nM and 139 nM, respectively. An even greater effect on the PB adjusted K103N activity was seen with two 6-fluoro-derivatives. Alkane-quinazolinone **120** and the alkynyl analog **115** had K103N values of 85 and 27 nM, respectively, while their PB adjusted K103N values were 357 and 891 nM, respectively. These examples underscore the importance of taking into consideration the protein binding profile of analogs, rather than solely looking at measured potency.

### INITIAL PHARMACOKINETIC EVALUATION

While iterative synthesis and testing were still ongoing, several compounds were selected for additional evaluation. Compounds **93** and **97** were chosen because of their outstanding resistance profile: 93 and 119 nM PB adj. K103N $IC_{90}$s, respectively (*Table 3.5*). The quinazolinone analog of efavirenz, compound **107**, was selected because it also had a good resistance profile (336 nM PB adj. K103N $IC_{90}$) and was structurally similar to efavirenz: the structural similarity was perceived to be an advantage since there were no overt toxicological issues associated with efavirenz and we expected the same to hold true for **107**.

Compounds **93**, **97** and **107** were synthesized on gram scale and submitted for resolution by chiral column HPLC. The active isomers were identified by screening both of the resolved enantiomers in the enzyme and antiviral assays, where activity was present in only one enantiomer (*Table 3.8*). The active

Table 3.8. ANTIVIRAL POTENCY FOR ENANTIOMERS OF **93, 97** AND **107**

| Compound | Enzyme $IC_{50}$ (nM) [31a] | Antiviral Activity Wild-Type $IC_{90}$ (nM) [31b] | Protein Binding Shift |
|---|---|---|---|
| **128** | $15 \pm 8$ | 1.6 | 9 |
| **129** | $1519 \pm 49$ | 229 | $ND^a$ |
| **DPC 961** | $31 \pm 8$ | $2.0 \pm 0.7$ | 18 |
| **130** | 267 | 34000 | $ND^a$ |
| **DPC 963** | $18 \pm 5$ | $1.3 \pm 0.6$ | 8.5 |
| **131** | 6600 | 101 | $ND^a$ |

$^a$ND = Not Determined.

isomers of **93, 107** and **97** were designated **128**, DPC 963 and DPC 961, respectively (*Figure 3.13*).

A mixture of **128**, DPC 961 and DPC 963 were administered orally to rhesus monkeys to rapidly obtain information regarding the pharmacokinetic properties of these molecules. Surprisingly, only DPC 961 and DPC 963 were found to be present in micromolar concentrations in plasma, while **128** was undetectable. Incubation of **128**, DPC 961 and DPC 963 in rhesus liver homogenate revealed that **128** was metabolized considerably faster than DPC 961 and DPC 963. The rapid metabolism of compounds without the cyclopropyl alkynyl group was also observed with benzoxazinones bearing the butyn-1-yl and 3-methylbutyn-1-yl alkynes, so the metabolism of **128** was not unique to quinazolinones. The recognition that simple alkyl chains appended onto the alkynes were rapidly metabolized in rhesus liver homogenate served to focus future SAR efforts. SAR work which was progressing simultaneously with the advancement of the quinazolinones revealed that olefin-containing benzox-

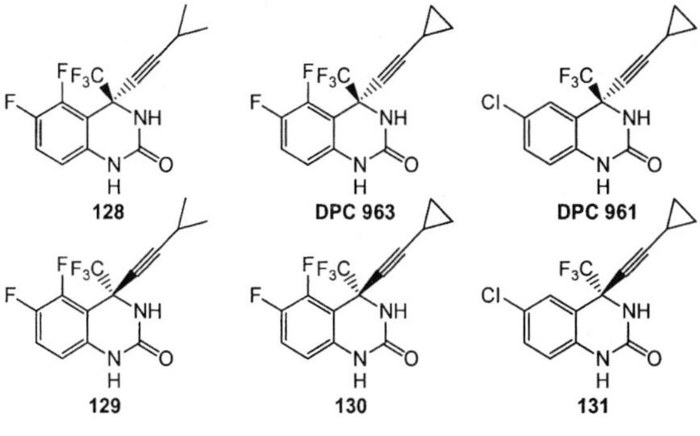

*Figure 3.13.*

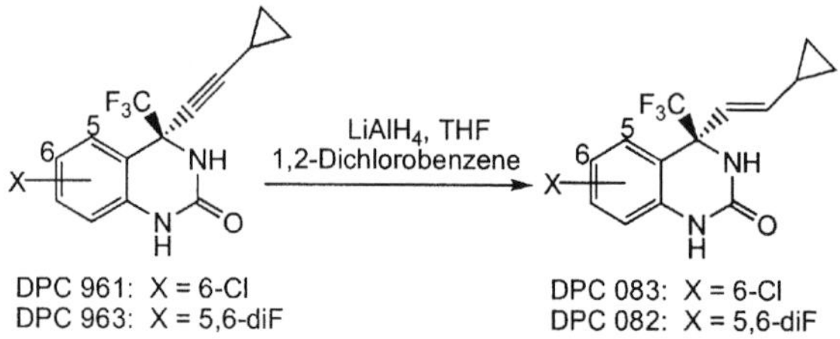

DPC 961: X = 6-Cl
DPC 963: X = 5,6-diF

DPC 083: X = 6-Cl
DPC 082: X = 5,6-diF

*Figure 3.14.*

azinones had lower protein binding. Such an improvement in protein binding upon removal of the alkynyl group from quinazolinones was also evident from the alkyl derivatives listed in *Table 3.6*. Therefore, DPC 961 and DPC 963 were reduced with lithium aluminum hydride (LAH) to provide the 6-chloro and 5,6-difluoro *trans*-olefins DPC 083 and DPC 082, respectively (*Figure 3.14*). The antiviral potency of the chiral quinazolinones DPC 082 and DPC 083 are given in *Table 3.9*. Indeed, DPC 082 and DPC 083 exhibited a substantial decrease in protein binding shift compared to their corresponding alkynes DPC 963 and DPC 961. The PB shift of the 6-chloro analog DPC 083 was approximately 4-times less than DPC 961, while a smaller two-fold difference was found for 5,6-difluoro analogs DPC 082 and DPC 963. No difference in the wild-type antiviral activity of the olefins and alkynes was observed.

ALTERNATE RING SYSTEM – EVALUATION OF 4,4'-DISUBSTITUTED
BENZOTHIADIAZINES

The success achieved with the quinazolinones prompted an evaluation of other related ring systems, a process that occurred simultaneously with the further exploration of the quinazolinones as described in previous and subsequent sections. A structural class closely related to the quinazolin-2(1*H*)-ones are the 1,3-*H*-2,1,3-benzothiadiazines [39]. The benzothiadiazines were interesting because they were a close structural analog of the quinazolinones and might

Table 3.9.   ANTIVIRAL POTENCY OF DPC 082 AND DPC 083

| Compound | Enzyme $IC_{50}$ (nM) [31a] | Antiviral Activity Wild-Type $IC_{90}$ (nM) [31b] | Protein Binding Shift |
|---|---|---|---|
| **DPC 082** | $27 \pm 2.3$ | $2.0 \pm 0.2$ | 4.2 |
| **DPC 083** | $23 \pm 1.7$ | $2.1 \pm 0.8$ | 4 |

present the substituents at the quaternary carbon center in approximately the same orientation as that obtained with the quinazolinones. The probability of success with these molecules was bolstered by reports in the literature describing other benzothiadiazines that possess activity as NNRTIs, albeit their inhibitory potency was marginal: MT-2 cell $EC_{50} = 9.5\,\mu M$ [40].

We found that treating 2-amino-5-chlorobenzonitrile (**132**) with cyclopropyl and isopropyl Grignard reagents at 45–50°C in THF provided the intermediate imine anions **133**, which were treated *in situ* with sulfuryl chloride to deliver **134a,b** (*Figure 3.15*). Prior to this research, there were no reports in the literature regarding the transformation of 1*H*-2,1,3-benzothiadiazines such as **134** into the 4,4-disubstituted derivative. The success achieved in the quinazolinone series in performing a similar transformation under Lewis acid catalysis provided a reasonable amount of confidence that the desired reaction could be accomplished. In the event, treating **134a,b** with lithiated acetylides in the presence of $BF_3 \cdot OEt_2$ afforded the desired adducts, albeit in modest yield (from 20% up to 56% yield for **142** and **136**, respectively). The corresponding 5,6-difluoro-4-trifluoromethyl benzothiadiazine analog **144** was prepared via a

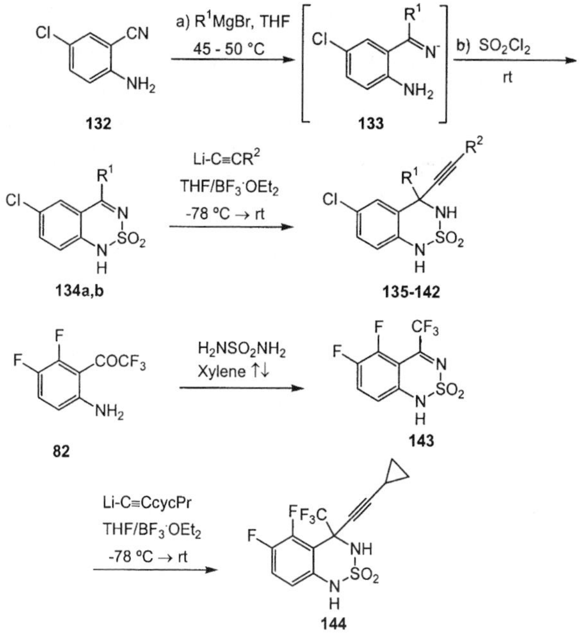

*Figure 3.15.*

Table 3.10.   BIOLOGICAL ACTIVITY OF BENZOTHIADIAZINES

| Compound | $R^1$ | $R^2$ | Enzyme $IC_{50}$ (nM) [31a] | Antiviral Activity $IC_{90}$ (nM) [31b] |
|---|---|---|---|---|
| DPC 961 | | | $31 \pm 8$ | $2.0 \pm 0.7$ |
| DPC 963 | | | $18 \pm 5$ | $1.3 \pm 0.6$ |
| Efavirenz | | | $47 \pm 25$ | $1.7 \pm 0.5$ |
| 135 | Cyclopropyl | i-Propyl | 4627 | 182 |
| 136 | Cyclopropyl | Cyclopropyl | 35,870 | 279 |
| 144 | $CF_3$ | Cyclopropyl | 24,667 | 284 |
| 137 | Cyclopropyl | Ethyl | Inactive | 611 |
| 138 | i-Propyl | i-Propyl | 24,137 | 643 |
| 139 | i-Propyl | Cyclopropyl | Inactive | 677 |
| 140 | i-Propyl | Ethyl | Inactive | 961 |
| 141 | Cyclopropyl | Phenyl | Inactive | Inactive |
| 142 | Cyclopropyl | 2-Pyridyl | Inactive | Inactive |

more traditional route which required heating **82** in xylenes at reflux with sulfamide to afford **143** [41]. The cyclopropylacetylide anion was added to **143**, as described for the addition to **134a,b**, to deliver **144**.

The benzothiadiazines had disappointing potency, with the most potent compound, **135**, having an $IC_{90} = 182$ nM (*Table 3.10*). It is clear that having either a cyclopropyl or trifluoromethyl group at $R^1$ (as in **135**, **136** and **144**) is needed for increased activity since compounds having an i-propyl group are substantially less active. The trifluoromethyl analog, **144**, was substantially less active in the antiviral assay than the corresponding 5,6-difluoro-quinazolinone analog, DPC 963: 279 nM versus 1.3 nM, respectively. Since the benzothiadiazines were substantially less potent than the most potent quinazolinones, such as DPC 961 and DPC 963, examination of this structural series was discontinued.

PREPARATION OF *N*-3 ALKYL QUINAZOLINONES

Examining the proposed mode of binding of the quinazolinones into the NNRTI binding pocket of RT indicated that there was the possibility of picking up favorable non-bonding interactions between the enzyme and groups appended to the *N*-3 nitrogen. Therefore, our attention turned to developing the chemistry needed to prepare *N*-3 alkyl quinazolinones. Eventually, three different approaches were developed to gain entry into these molecules. Two of these approaches, which utilize a common intermediate, are shown in *Figure 3.16*. The first method involves reacting ketones **60** and **82** with alkyl isocyanates to provide aminols **145a, b** (R = methyl or ethyl). Another route to the aminols, which avoids the use of isocyanates, involved exposing

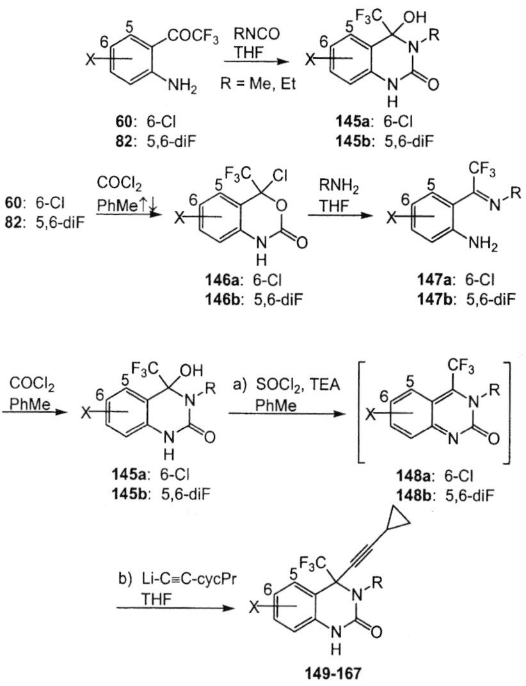

*Figure 3.16.*

chlorobenzoxazinones **146a,b**, obtained from **60** and **82** upon treatment with phosgene in toluene at reflux [34], to an excess amount of amine in THF at 0°C to deliver imines **147a,b**. The stable, purifiable imines were then treated with a solution of phosgene in toluene to yield the *N*-3 alkyl aminols **145a,b** (R ≠ methyl or ethyl).

Dissolving aminols **145a,b** (either obtained directly from **60** and **82** or from **146a,b**) in toluene containing triethylamine and cooling to 0°C followed by the dropwise addition of thionyl chloride gave the intermediate "tetraenes" **148a,b** to which cyclopropyl acetylide was added to afford the desired alkyl quinazolinones **149–167** [42].

Several analogs were also prepared that explored the effects of a polar, hydrogen bond acceptor/donor at the *N*-3 position. Compounds **159** and **160** were converted into the corresponding amides **168** and **169** (*Figure 3.17*) [18]. Exposing **146a** to *t*-butyldimethylsilyl-protected ethanolamine **170** [44] gave **171**, which was converted into silyl ether **172** via the protocol shown in *Figure 3.16*, involving an intermediate "tetraene". Desilylation of TBS-ether **172** with TBAF gave **173**. Alcohol **173** also underwent a Swern oxidation to

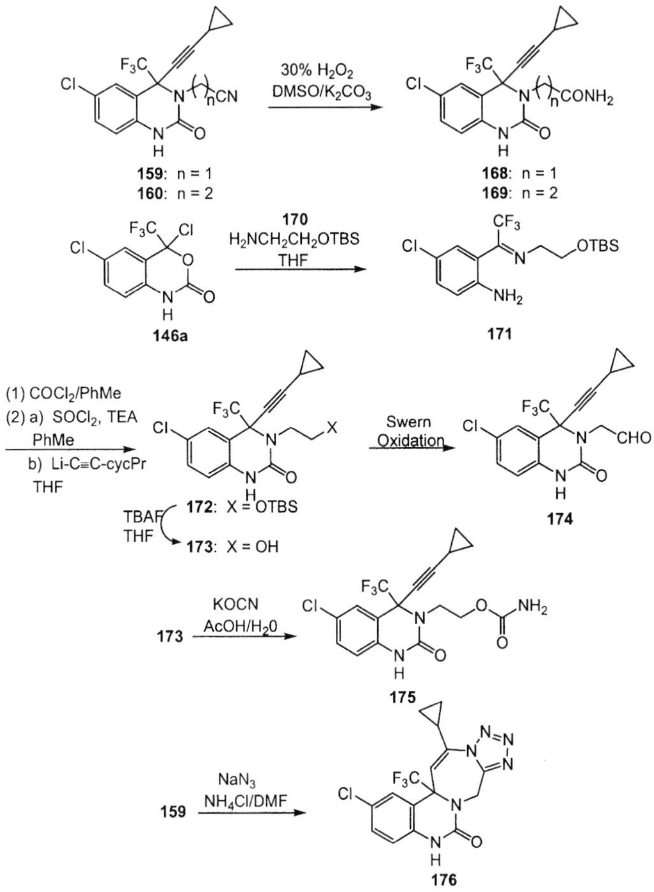

*Figure 3.17.*

provide aldehyde **174**. Carbamate **175** was obtained from **173** upon treatment with potassium cyanate in a mixture of acetic acid and water. We also envisioned utilizing the nitrile functionality present in **159** as a handle to introduce a tetrazole ring.

Heating **159** with a mixture of sodium azide and ammonium chloride in dimethylformamide (DMF) provided the expected tetrazole, which subsequently cyclized onto the cyclopropyl alkynyl group to yield the unique tetracycle **176**.

Our experience with the quinazolinones had indicated that *trans*-olefins had unique properties, such as decreased protein binding. Because the protein binding was often extensive with the *N*-3 alkyl derivatives (see compounds **150** and **151** in *Table 3.11*), we needed a rapid, versatile synthetic approach to the *N*-3 alkyl *trans*-olefin quinazolinones. The process that we found to provide the molecules of interest is shown in *Figure 3.18*. Ketones **60** and **82** could be converted into their corresponding PMB-protected derivatives **177a,b** upon treatment with *p*-methoxybenzyl alcohol containing *p*-toluenesulfonic acid in a solution of acetonitrile [45]. Heating potassium cyanate with a solution of **177a** or **b** in an acetic acid/water mixture gave aminols **178a,b**, which were subsequently dehydrated by heating at reflux in toluene (for **178a**) or xylenes (for **178b**) to yield ketimines

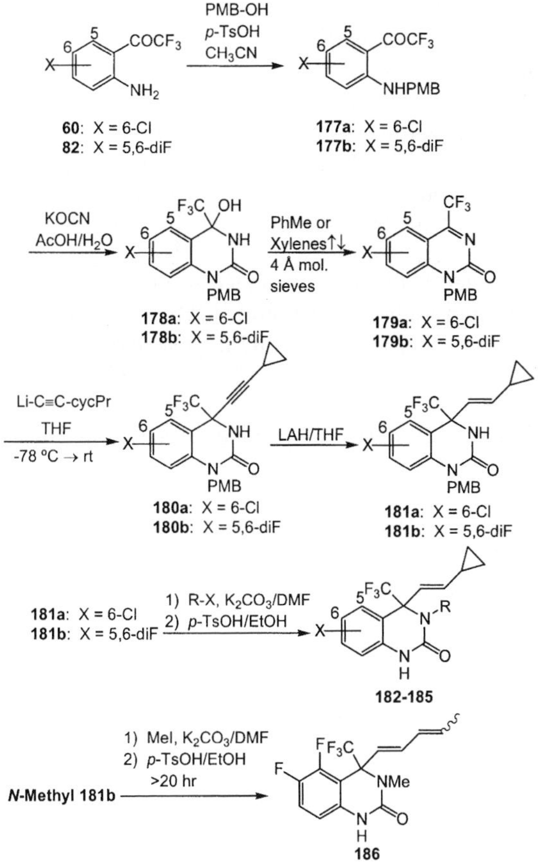

*Figure 3.18.*

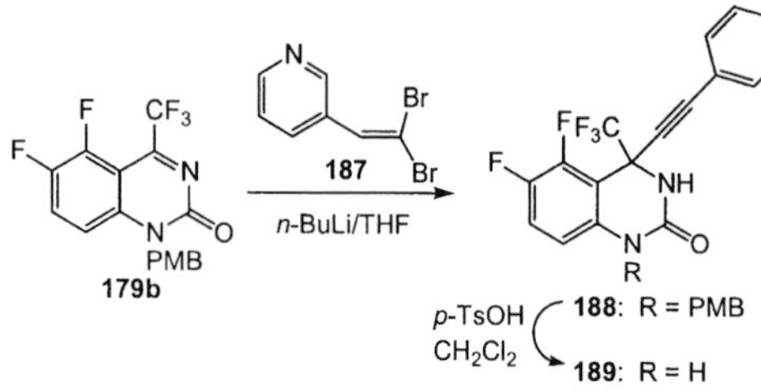

*Figure 3.19.*

**179a,b.** Addition of lithiated acetylides to **179a,b** proceeded uneventfully, without the need for the addition of boron trifluoride etherate, to yield $N$-1 protected quinazolinones **180a,b**. Directed LAH reduction of the alkynes yielded *trans*-olefins **181a,b**. The $N$-3 alkyl group was then incorporated into **181a,b** upon treatment with an alkyl halide in dimethylformamide (DMF) containing potassium carbonate, and the PMB-group was removed using $p$-toluenesulfonic acid in ethanol to provide the desired final products **182–185**. It was found that the conditions used for PMB removal from $N$-methyl **181b** were critical. If the reaction went too long, the only product isolated was diene **186**.

The PMB-protected ketimine also proved useful in the preparation of a 3-pyridylacetylene quinazolinone. Ketimine **179b** was treated with the alkyne generated *in situ* from dibromo-olefin **187** to yield **188** (*Figure 3.19*) [34]. The PMB-group was subsequently removed using $p$-toluenesulfonic acid to provide quinazolinone **189**.

The biological activity for the compounds prepared in *Figure 3.15* through *Figure 3.19* are exhibited in *Table 3.11*. The incorporation of polar groups onto $N$-3 gave compounds with marginal activity toward wild-type virus and poor activity toward K103N (**168, 169** and **173**). Large alkyl and phenethyl groups on $N$-3 provided compounds that had a similarly disappointing profile exhibiting poor antiviral efficacy (**161–167**). Small alkyl groups provided the best activity, with good activity against K103N being achieved with $N$-3 substituted with methyl, ethyl, $i$-propyl, cyclopropyl, or cyclopropyl methyl groups (compounds **149–156**).

### PREPARATION OF QUINAZOLINTHIONES

Having identified potent quinazolinones, we turned our attention to discovering compounds with improved potency against mutant viral forms. The increased potency of the quinazolinthiones demonstrated in the early work by Merck prompted us to investigate trifluoromethyl-containing quinazolinthiones [21a].

Table 3.11. BIOLOGICAL ACTIVITY OF DIFFERENTIALLY SUBSTITUTED
QUINAZOLINONES

| Compound | X | R | Enzyme $IC_{50}$ (nM) [31a] | Wild-Type Antiviral Activity [31b] | PB Adj. Wild Type Activity | K103N Antiviral Acivity | PB Fold Shift |
|---|---|---|---|---|---|---|---|
| **Alkynes** | | | | | | | |
| **Efavirenz** | | | $47 \pm 25$ | $1.7 \pm 0.5$ | 28 | $64 \pm 24$ | 16.5 |
| **149** | 6-Cl | $CH_3$ | $36 \pm 10$ | 9 | 630 | 64 | 70 |
| **150** | 5,6-diF | $CH_3$ | $49 \pm 8$ | 8 | 536 | 15 | 67 |
| **151** | 6-Cl | $CH_2CH_3$ | $93 \pm 25$ | 13 | 117 | 22 | 9 |
| **152** | 5,6-diF | $CH_2CH_3$ | $197 \pm 55$ | 9 | | 20 | $ND^a$ |
| **153** | 6-Cl | Cyclopropyl | $419 \pm 254$ | 20 | 1218 | 48 | 6 |
| **154** | 5,6-diF | Cyclopropyl | $49 \pm 8$ | 8 | | 15 | $ND^a$ |
| **155** | 5,6-diF | $CH_2cycPr$ | $255 \pm 33$ | 14 | | 22 | $ND^a$ |
| **156** | 6-Cl | $CH(CH_3)_2$ | $465 \pm 133$ | 24 | | 39 | $ND^a$ |
| **157** | 6-Cl | $CH_2CH(OEt)_2$ | $1550 \pm 44$ | 162 | | 3946 | $ND^a$ |
| **158** | 6-Cl | $CH_2CH_2OEt$ | $192 \pm 100$ | 20 | 380 | 259 | 19 |
| **159** | 6-Cl | $CH_2CN$ | $71 \pm 5$ | 10 | | 147 | $ND^a$ |
| **160** | 6-Cl | $CH_2CH_2CN$ | $130 \pm 50$ | 11 | | $ND^a$ | $ND^a$ |
| **161** | 6-Cl | Phenethyl | $1491 \pm 269$ | 153 | | $ND^a$ | $ND^a$ |
| **162** | 6-Cl | (2-FluoroPh)ethyl | $1508 \pm 162$ | 320 | | $ND^a$ | $ND^a$ |
| **163** | 6-Cl | (4-MeOPh)ethyl | 1502 | 189 | | $ND^a$ | $ND^a$ |
| **164** | 6-Cl | (3,4-DiMeOPh)ethyl | $711 \pm 186$ | 123 | | $ND^a$ | $ND^a$ |
| **165** | 6-Cl | (2-MeOPh)ethyl | 1758 | 668 | | $ND^a$ | $ND^a$ |
| **166** | 6-Cl | (3-ChloroPh)ethyl | 7019 | 1103 | | $ND^a$ | $ND^a$ |
| **167** | 6-Cl | (3-MeOPh)ethyl | 2600 | ND | | $ND^a$ | $ND^a$ |
| **168** | 6-Cl | $CH_2CONH_2$ | $1523 \pm 199$ | 59 | | 4570 | $ND^a$ |
| **169** | 6-Cl | $CH_2CH_2CONH_2$ | $270 \pm 81$ | 23 | | 855 | $ND^a$ |
| **173** | 6-Cl | $CH_2CH_2OH$ | $141 \pm 46$ | 11 | | 307 | $ND^a$ |
| **174** | 6-Cl | $CH_2CHO$ | $495 \pm 237$ | 21 | | $ND^a$ | $ND^a$ |
| **175** | 6-Cl | $CH_2CH_2OCONH_2$ | $190 \pm 45$ | 10 | | $ND^a$ | $ND^a$ |
| **176** | 6-Cl | See *Figure 3.17* | $553 \pm 33$ | 10 | | 252 | $ND^a$ |
| **189** | 5,6-diF | See *Figure 3.19* | $39 \pm 7$ | 8.5 | 60 | 54 | 7 |
| **Olefins** | | | | | | | |
| **182** | 6-Cl | Ethyl | $122 \pm 88$ | 9.3 | 102 | 16 | 11 |
| **183** | 5,6-diF | $CH_2cycPr$ | $241 \pm 169$ | 14 | 266 | 20 | 19 |
| **184** | 6-Cl | $CH_2cycPr$ | $191 \pm 56$ | 30 | 510 | 27 | 17 |
| **185** | 5,6-diF | $CH_3$ | $56 \pm 26$ | 6.6 | 106 | $ND^a$ | 16 |

$^a$ND = Not Determined.

Improvements in potency achieved through the use of a thiourea have also been observed in the TIBO [46] and PETT [47] series of NNRTIs.

It was initially perceived that entry into the quinazolinthiones would be relatively straight-forward: replace potassium cyanate with potassium thiocyanate or a suitably derivatized alkyl isothiocyanate and follow the synthetic route delineated in *Figure 3.11*. In fact, differences in the reactivity between 6-chloro-and 5,6-difluoro-containing *N*-alkyl quinazolinthione intermediates resulted in the development of different synthetic approaches to the desired final products. As point of fact, methyl isothiocyanate reacted cleanly with **60** and **82** to provide *N*-methyl aminols **190a,b** (*Figure 3.20*). Generating the "tetraene" intermediates **191a,b** and addition of lithiated cyclopropylacetylide, as described in *Figure 3.17*, afforded only the desired 6-chloro-containing quinazolinthione **192**, with none of the desired adduct arising from **19lb**. For this reason, an alternate route to the 5,6-difluoro-containing compounds was sought. Eventually we found that **150** could be converted into thiourea **193** by phosphorus oxychloride. This gave an intermediate iminoyl chloride that was concentrated to dryness but not isolated, followed by heating at reflux with thiourea in ethanol [46b]. *N*-Cyclopropylmethyl, 6-chloro-thiourea **194** was prepared from urea **153** in a similar fashion.

The preparation of thioureas not having a *N*-3 alkyl group was difficult. For instance, the addition of alkynyl lithium reagents to thioketimines **l95a,b** resulted in a complex reaction mixture and was not investigated further (*Figure 3.21*). A solution to this problem was found by converting **180a,b** to the iminoyl chlorides with phosphorus oxychloride, concentrating and heating at reflux with thiourea in ethanol. This procedure delivered the *N*-3 unsubstituted

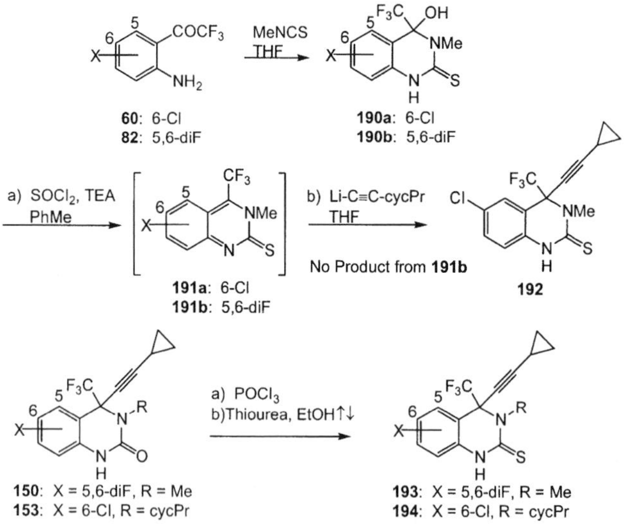

Figure 3.20.

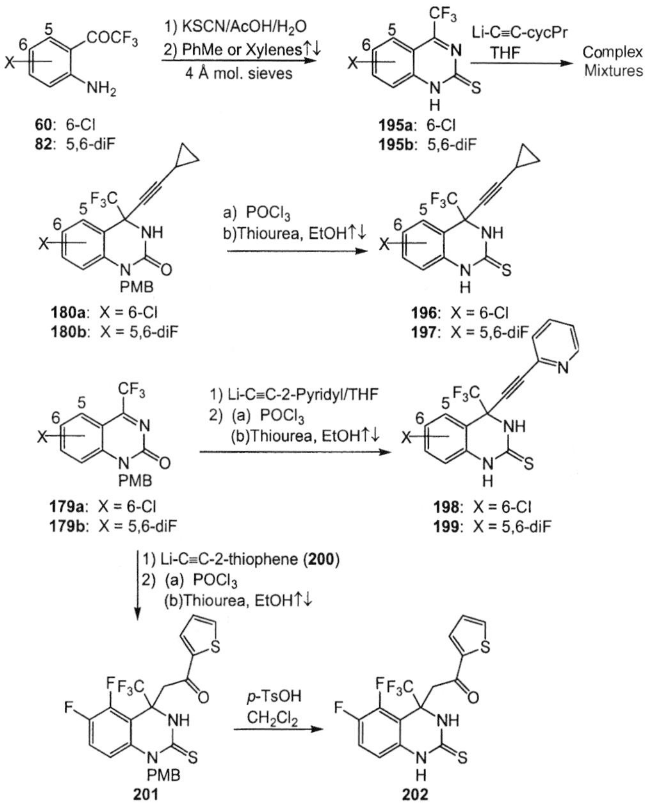

*Figure 3.21.*

thioureas **196** and **197**. Presumably the PMB-group was cleaved during the workup by acid generated from residual POCl₃. The 2-pyridyl alkyne analogs **198** and **199** were prepared in an analogous manner from PMB-protected ketimines **179a,b**. However, addition of lithiated 2-ethynylthiophene (**200**) to **179b** afforded the PMB-protected ketone **201**, after treatment with phosphorus oxychloride and thiourea. The PMB-group was removed from **201** upon treatment with *p*-toluenesulfonic acid to yield **202**.

The thiourea *trans*-olefin **203** was obtained by reducing **197** with lithium aluminum hydride (*Figure 3.22*). The *N*-methyl analog of **203** was obtained by treating the iminoyl chloride obtained from **185** with thiourea in hot ethanol to afford **204**. The same reaction sequence was performed on diene **186** to provide the *N*-methyl diene analog **205**.

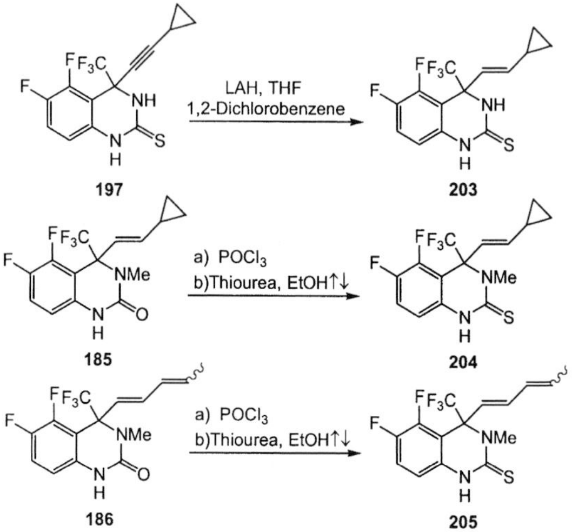

*Figure 3.22.*

The biological activity of all of the compounds prepared in *Figures 3.20* through *Figure 3.22* is shown in *Table 3.12*. Several thioureas exhibited low nanomolar against the K103N mutant, and were the most potent compounds against this RT mutation. The 5,6-difluoroquinazolinthiones **193** and **197** had potency against the K103N mutant which was comparable to their activity against wild-type virus: 7.2 and 4.8 nM for **193** and 2.6 and 4.2 nM for **197** against wild-type and K103N, respectively. The corresponding 6-chloroquinazolinthiones **192** and **196** possessed similar potency against K103N as **193** and **197**.

## IDENTIFICATION OF DRUG CANDIDATES

Several racemic compounds with desirable antiviral properties required the separation of the enantiomers. The first compounds chosen have already been presented: DPC 082, DPC 083, DPC 961 and DPC 963. The measured potency of DPC 082, DPC 083, DPC 961 and DPC 963 against several clinically significant HIV-1 RT mutants are given in *Table 3.13*. All of the compounds had HIV-1 RF measured potency that was very similar to efavirenz, with the differences between the compounds being evident in their respective resistance profiles against the several single and double mutant viral forms. For instance, DPC 082, DPC 083, DPC 961 and DPC 963 were all about ten-fold more potent

Table 3.12. BIOLOGICAL ACTIVITY OF QUINAZOLINTHIONES

| Compound | Y | X | R | Enzyme $IC_{50}$ (nM) [31a] | Wild-Type Antiviral Activity [31b] | $IC_{90}$ (nM) PB Adj. Wild Type Activity | K103N Antiviral Activity | PB Fold Shift |
|---|---|---|---|---|---|---|---|---|
| **Efavirenz** | | | | 47±25 | 1.7±0.5 | 28 | 64±24 | 16.5 |
| 192 | NMe | 6-Cl | C≡C-cycPr | 219±69 | 6.7 | | 10±1 | ND[a] |
| 193 | NMe | 5,6-diF | C≡C-cycPr | 140±18 | 7.2 | | 4.8±3 | ND[a] |
| 194 | NcycPr | 6-Cl | C≡C-cycPr | 877±333 | 19 | 171 | ND[a] | 9 |
| 196 | NH | 6-Cl | C≡C-cycPr | 174±30 | 3.3 | 76 | 8.5 | 23 |
| 197 | NH | 5,6-diF | C≡C-cycPr | 121±57 | 2.6 | 17 | 4.2±3 | 6.5 |
| 198 | NH | 6-Cl | C≡C-2-Pyridyl | 1817±714 | 139 | | ND[a] | ND[a] |
| 199 | NH | 5,6-diF | C≡C-2-Pyridyl | 7499±313 | 244 | | ND[a] | ND[a] |
| 202 | NH | 5,6-diF | CH₂CO-2-thienyl | 146±24 | 10 | 50 | >357 | 5 |
| 203 | NH | 5,6-diF | CH=CH-cycPr | 196±56 | 5.1 | | 18 | ND[a] |
| 204 | NMe | 5,6-diF | CH=CH-cycPr | 329±111 | 7.8 | 86 | ND[a] | 11 |
| 205 | NMe | 5,6-diF | CH=CHCH=CHMe | 366±241 | 8.3 | 83 | ND[a] | 10 |

[a]ND = Not Determined.

Table 3.13. RESISTANCE PROFILE OF DPC 082, DPC 083, DPC 961 AND DPC 963

| | Measured Potency $IC_{90}$ (nM) | | | | | |
|---|---|---|---|---|---|---|
| Compound | Wild-Type (HIV-1 RF) | K103N | L100I | K103N-V108I | K103N-P225H | K103N-L100I |
| DPC 082 | $2.0 \pm 0.2$ | $21 \pm 9.2$ | $5.9 \pm 3.8$ | $22. \pm 140$ | $180 \pm 29$ | $550 \pm 400$ |
| DPC 083 | $2.1 \pm 0.8$ | $27 \pm 11$ | $11 \pm 6.8$ | $90 \pm 6.6$ | $140 \pm 92$ | $1690 \pm 160$ |
| DPC 961 | $2.0 \pm 0.7$ | $10 \pm 3.2$ | $13 \pm 7.9$ | $38 \pm 4$ | $73 \pm 18$ | $1100 \pm 160$ |
| DPC 963 | $1.3 \pm 0.6$ | $11 \pm 4.8$ | $8.0 \pm 5.7$ | $34 \pm 5.4$ | $46 \pm 2.2$ | $890 \pm 90$ |
| Efavirenz | $1.7 \pm 0.5$ | $64 \pm 30$ | $120 \pm 30$ | $240 \pm 68$ | $310 \pm 130$ | $7300 \pm 5000$ |

against the L100I mutant than efavirenz. The alkynes DPC 961 and DPC 963 were about six-fold more potent against K103N than efavirenz, while the olefins DPC 082 and DPC 083 were about three-times more active. A major improvement in the resistance profile was evident when the K103N-containing double mutants were examined. The alkynes DPC 961 and DPC 963 were dramatically more effective in inhibiting K103N-V108I and K103N-P225H than efavirenz. The 6-chloro-olefin, DPC 083, performed well against the double mutants, but the measured potency was above that of the alkynes. The 5,6-difluoroolefin, DPC 082, was the least effective compound against the two more common double mutants, but it had the best measured potency against the rare K103N-L100I mutant.

Throughout the discovery process, the impact of protein binding had been estimated from the shift assay. Although the shift assay was useful for rapid comparisons between closely related analogs, it did not provide a quantitative value for free drug levels. Since only free (unbound) drug is available to diffuse into the cell for binding to the intracellular target, methods to accurately determine free drug fraction were developed. Equilibrium dialysis and ultrafiltration coupled with LC/MS can be used to measure trace quantities of free drug in equilibrium with plasma proteins. Because tissue culture medium also contains small quantities of plasma proteins (10–20% fetal calf serum is typically utilized in tissue culture experiments), the free fraction present in this biological mileau was also determined. The free drug levels for DPC 961, DPC 963, DPC 083 and DPC 082 in human serum or tissue culture medium are shown in *Table 3.14*, along with measured values for efavirenz. Because efavirenz is extensively bound to serum proteins, a range of values reflecting several different assays is shown. The quinazolinones are less highly protein bound than efavirenz. In fact there is up to ten-times more free drug available in human plasma with the quinazolinones than for efavirenz.

We defined a parameter designated intrinsic potency as the free drug concentration capable of 90% suppression of virus replication. Intrinsic potency

Table 3.14. FREE DRUG LEVELS OF DPC 082, DPC 083, DPC 961 AND DPC 963

| Compound | % Free Drug In Tissue Culture Medium | % Free Drug In Human Plasma |
|---|---|---|
| DPC 082 | 53 | 3.0 |
| DPC 083 | 39 | 2.0 |
| DPC 961 | 31 | 1.5 |
| DPC 963 | 37 | 2.8 |
| Efavirenz | 27.2 | 0.21–0.54 |

thus allows a comparison of the in vitro antiviral activity in the context of protein binding. To calculate the intrinsic potency, the percent of free drug in tissue culture medium (the value from *Table 3.14*) was multiplied by the measured potency obtained in *Table 3.13* and these values are displayed in *Table 3.15*. All of the compounds selected for development have intrinsic potencies below efavirenz against all of the mutant virus' tested, except for DPC 082. Development of DPC 082 continued since it possessed excellent intrinsic potency against the K103N-L100I mutant.

DPC 082, DPC 083, DPC 961 and DPC 963 were combined and dosed orally in rhesus monkeys (10 mg/kg) and individually in chimpanzees (2 mg/kg) with the pharmacokinetic properties listed in *Table 3.16*. To directly compare the rhesus and chimpanzee pharmacokinetic data, the measured 24-hour levels in the chimp at 2 mg/kg were multiplied by 5 to reflect a 10 mg/kg dose. The measured serum protein binding for each compound (*Table 3.14*) was then used to calculate the free drug at 24 hours in the chimpanzee. The $t_{1/2}$ of the 6-chloroquinazolinones DPC 083 and DPC 961 were longer in rhesus and chimpanzee than for the corresponding 5,6-difluoro derivatives DPC 082 and DPC 963. In fact, DPC 083 had $t_{1/2} > 85$ hours in chimpanzee. The half life

Table 3.15. FREE DRUG (INTRINSIC) POTENCY OF DPC 082, DPC 083, DPC 961 AND DPC 963

| Compound | Wild-Type (HIV-1 RF) | K103N | L100I | K103N-V108I | K103N-P225H | K103N-L100I |
|---|---|---|---|---|---|---|
| | *Intrinsic Potency $IC_{90}$ (nM)* | | | | | |
| DPC 082 | 1.1 | 11 | 3 | 117 | 95 | 292 |
| DPC 083 | 0.8 | 11 | 4 | 35 | 55 | 660 |
| DPC 961 | 0.6 | 3.1 | 4 | 12 | 23 | 340 |
| DPC 963 | 0.5 | 4.0 | 3 | 13 | 17 | 330 |
| Efavirenz | 0.5 | 17 | 33 | 65 | 84 | 1990 |

Table 3.16.  PHARMACOKINETIC PROFILE OF DPC 082, DPC 083, DPC 961 AND DPC 963

| | | Concn ($\mu M$) at 24 h in[a]: | | | |
|---|---|---|---|---|---|
| Compound | Rhesus monkey | Chimpanzee (2 mg/kg data normalized to 10 mg/kg) | $t_{1/2}$ (h) Rhesus | $t_{1/2}$ (h) Chimpanzee | Free Drug Concn (nM) at 24 h in Chimpanzee |
| DPC 082 | 0.64 | 4.7 | 5.9 | 14.2 | 141 |
| DPC 083 | 6.84 | 7.6 | 24 | 85.7 | 152 |
| DPC 961 | 0.38 | 12.7 | 4.8 | 76.0 | 191 |
| DPC 963 | 0.22 | 6.2 | 4.8 | 19.6 | 174 |
| Efavirenz | 0.36 | 2.7 | ND | ND[a] | 6−15 |

[a]ND = Not Determined.

values observed in the chimpanzee for all 4 compounds are consistant with a once-daily dosing regimen. The lower protein binding of the quinazolinones played a significant role in the free drug concentration at 24 hours: there was between 9 and 31-times more drug available at trough plasma levels (assuming once-daily dosing) for the quinazolinones than for efavirenz.

As detailed in the introduction, our primary objective was to find drugs that would be predicted to have blood levels high enough to cover relevant mutant viral forms, and to accomplish this with once-daily dosing. For this goal to be met, the trough levels of free drug must exceed the intrinsic potency for the clinically relevant mutant variants of HIV. This calculation was performed using the free drug plasma levels obtained from chimpanzees. In *Table 3.17*, the trough levels of free drug are divided by the $IC_{90}$ of the free drug (intrinsic potency) to provide a ratio. A value $>1$ indicates that the amount of free drug available after 24 hours is greater than the free drug $IC_{90}$. A value in *Table 3.17* $>1$ would be indicative of the ability of a drug to suppress viral replication of that particular form of HIV.

Table 3.17.  RATIO OF 24 HOUR FREE DRUG LEVELS TO INTRINSIC POTENCY VALUES

| | Ratio of trough level of free drug in chimpanzees/$IC_{90}$ of free drug | | | | |
|---|---|---|---|---|---|
| Compound | Wild-Type | K103M | K103N-V108I | K103N-P225H | K103N-L100I |
| DPC 082 | 128 | 13 | 1.2 | 1.5 | 0.5 |
| DPC 083 | 190 | 14 | 4.3 | 2.8 | 0.2 |
| DPC 961 | 318 | 62 | 16 | 8.3 | 0.6 |
| DPC 963 | 348 | 44 | 13 | 10 | 0.5 |
| Efavirenz | 12−30 | 0.4−0.9 | 0.09−0.2 | 0.07−0.2 | 0.003−0.008 |

As shown in *Table 3.17*, the ratio of free drug at trough relative to the K103N IC$_{90}$ ranged from 13- to 62-fold. In contrast, efavirenz free drug level approaches unity for the K103N mutant, but does not exceed the concentration required. Furthermore, all four quinazolinones would be expected to provide sufficient blood levels at trough to provide coverage for two of the most common K103N-containing double mutants, K103N-V108I and K103N-P225H. The least common double mutant, K103N-L100I, escaped coverage at trough by all four compounds as evidenced values less than 1.

Meanwhile, in attempts to find compounds with an even better overall profile, we examined the thiourea and *N*-3 alkyl series of compounds. Two *N*-3 alkyl, **153** and **183**, and two thiourea, **193** and **197**, derivatives were selected for further evaluation because of their excellent resistance profile against a panel of clinically significant mutant forms of HIV-1 (*Table 3.18*). The *trans*-olefin derivative **183** had the lowest K103N-L100I IC$_{90}$ for any of the quinazolinones and -thiones tested. The protein binding shift data for **153** and **197** suggested that these compounds may have significant free fraction in human plasma: the PB fold shift was 6 and 6.5 for **153** and **197**, respectively (data from Table and Table).

Chiral HPLC resolution of **153**, **183**, **193** and **197** provided the active enantiomers **206**, **207**, **208** and **209**, respectively (*Figure 3.23*). The biological data for the active enantiomers is in *Table 3.19*.

Compounds **206** through **209** were dosed orally in rhesus monkeys and the pharmacokinetic profiles are shown in *Table 3.20*. Unfortunately, it was found that the *N*-3 alkyl compounds were extremely highly protein bound in human plasma and the protein binding fold shift values were not predictive of the free fraction of drug for highly lipophilic compounds: **206** had less than 0.2% free drug [38]. For this reason, the free drug concentration at 24 hours for **206** was

Table 3.18.   IMPROVED RESISTANCE PROFILE OF *N*-3 ALKYL QUINAZOLINONES AND – THIONES

| | *Antiviral Activity IC$_{90}$ (nM)* | | | | | | |
|---|---|---|---|---|---|---|---|
| *Compound* | *Wild-Type (HIV-1 RF)* | *K103N* | *G190S* | *K103N-V108I* | *K103N-P225H* | *K103N-K101E* | *K103N-L100I* |
| **151** | 20 | 48 | 71 | 144 | 197 | ND$^a$ | 214 |
| **183** | 14 | 20 | 51 | 91 | 71 | ND$^a$ | 99 |
| **193** | 7 | 4.8 ± 3 | 8.7 | 8.5 ± 1.4 | 18 ± 8 | 32 | 153 |
| **197** | 2.6 | 4.2 ± 3 | 11 | 6.0 ± 6.4 | 26 ± 6.4 | 33 | 292 |
| **Efavirenz** | 1.7 ± 0.5 | 64 ± 30 | | 240 ± 68 | 310 ± 13 | | 7300 ± 5000 |

$^a$ND = Not Determined.

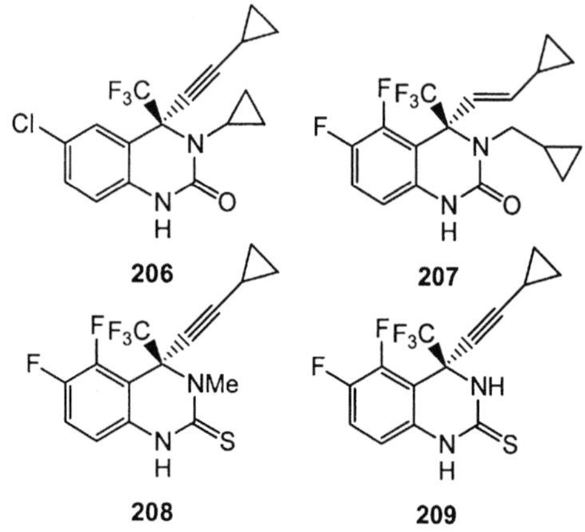

**206** **207**

**208** **209**

*Figure 3.23.*

unacceptable. Thiourea **209** was dosed in rhesus monkeys, and very low and variable blood levels were observed. The low blood levels were thought to be due to poor aqueous solubility and not due to poor cellular permeability since Caco-2 permeation measurements, using 5% N, N-dimethylacetamide (DMAC) as a solubilizing agent, resulted in measurable amounts of drug: 0.3 mM at pH 7.4, and 0.4 mM at pH 5.0. Papp values for **209** were 65 and $252 \times 10^{-6}$ cm/sec, at pH 7.4 and 5.0, respectively. Thus we focused upon developing DPC 082, DPC 083, DPC 961 and DPC 963 after the disappointing pharmacokinetic profiles of **206** through **209**.

Table 3.19.  BIOLOGICAL ACTIVITY OF RESOLVED QUINAZOLINONES
AND – THIONES

| Compound | Enzyme $IC_{50}$ (nM) [31a] | Wild-Type Antiviral Activity $IC_{90}$ (nM) [31b] |
|---|---|---|
| **206** | $83 \pm 51$ | 8 |
| **207** | $157 \pm 60$ | ND[a] |
| **208** | $115 \pm 41$ | ND[a] |
| **209** | $217 \pm 31$ | 2 |
| **Efavirenz** | $47 \pm 25$ | $1.7 \pm 0.5$ |

[a]ND = Not Determined.

Table 3.20. PHARMACOKINETIC PROFILE OF *N*-3 ALKYL QUINAZOLINONES
AND – THIONES

| Compound | Rhesus monkey Concn (µM) at 24 h in[a] | $t_{1/2}$ (h) | Free Drug Concn (nM) at 24 h | % Free Drug in Human Plasma |
|---|---|---|---|---|
| 206 | | 52[b] | 22 | <0.2 |
| 207 | | | 0 | |
| 208 | | | | |
| 209 | 0 | 2.6[c], 9.8[d], 5.3[e] | | ND |
| Efavirenz | 0.36 | ND | 6–15 | 0.21–0.54 |

[a]The drug was administered to rhesus monkeys orally at 10 mg/kg. Data for chimpanzees, which were given 2 mg/kg, are extrapolated from data for rhesus monkeys. [b]The $t_{1/2}$ is for chimpanzee. [c]The $t_{1/2}$ is for rhesus monkey dosed in methylcellulose. [d]The $t_{1/2}$ is for rhesus monkey dosed in DMAC/tween/PG. [e]The $t_{1/2}$ is for chimpanzee.

## CONCLUSION

A versatile approach to highly functionalized quinazolinones was developed that enabled the independent derivatization of the aromatic ring, incorporation of various groups pendant to the quaternary carbon and substitution of the *N*-3 nitrogen with a variety of hydrophobic and hydrophilic groups. Furthermore, several synthetic approaches were developed that enabled the preparation of thiourea derivatives. Thorough evaluation of these compounds has indicated that it is critical to not only evaluate the measured potency, but to also consider the free drug concentration when comparing compounds. The failure to do so with the quinazolinones would probably have resulted in not initially recognizing that these NNRTIs represented a significant improvement over all existing drug therapies. The pharmacokinetic parameters and resistance profile observed for DPC 082, DPC 083, DPC 961 and DPC 963 were deemed sufficient to warrant advancing all four compounds into Phase I clinical trials. The Phase I data for DPC 961 has been reported [48] and Phase II data for DPC 083 has been reported [49]. Based on these encouraging data, DPC 961 and DPC 083 will be examined in Phase II trials in HIV-positive subjects as part of a combination therapy regimen. If adequate exposure and tolerability can be demonstrated, DPC 961 or DPC 083 could provide important additions to the AIDS therapy armamentarium, especially for patients with NNRTI mutations.

## ACKNOWLEDGEMENTS

The following group of researchers was responsible for providing critical data that enabled the rapid development of the DuPont Pharmaceuticals Company non-nucleoside reverse transcriptase project: Soo Ko, Senliang Pan, Kristen J. Kresge, Susan Jeffrey, Lee T. Bacheler, Ronald M. Klabe, David Crist, Sharon Diamond, Chii-Ming Lai, Sena Garber, Beverly C. Cordova, Shelley Rabel, Jo Anne Saye, Stephen P. Adams, George L. Trainor, Paul S. Anderson, and Susan K. Erickson-Viitanen.

## REFERENCES

1   The White House, Office of the Press Secretary: A National Security Strategy for a New Century, January 5, 2000.

2   Kilby, J. M.; Saag, M. S. In *Manual of HIV Therapeutics*, Powderly, W. G., Ed.; Lippincott-Raven: New York, 1997: p. 1.

3   Ho, D. D.; Neumann, A. U.; Perelson, A. S.; Chen, W.; Leonard, J. M.; Markowitz, M. *Nature* **1995**, *373*, 123–6.

4   Levy, J. A. *Microbiol. Rev.* **1993**, *57*, 183.

5   Jonckheere, H.; Anné, J.; De Clercq, E. *Med. Res. Rev.* **2000**, *20*, 129.

6   The reader interested in the history of the discovery of NRTIs is directed to: De Clercq, E. *J. Med. Chem.* **1995**, *38*, 2491.

7   (a) Nusbaum, N. J.; Joseph, P. E. *Cell Biol.* **1996**, *15*, 363. (b) Kakuda, T. N. *Clin. Ther.* **2000**, *22*, 685; (c) Moyle, G. *Drug Saf.* **2000**, *23*, 467.

8   For a discussion regarding the biochemical basis for the development of resistance toward NRTIs, see: Götte, M.; Wainberg, M. A. *Drug Resist. Updates* **2000**, *3*, 30.

9   Information obtained from package inserts for indinavir (taken without food), ritonavir (taken with food to increase absorption), saquinavir (taken with food to increase absorption).

10  Information on adverse events can be found in the package inserts or on the internet at http://www.aidsmeds.com/lessons/Drug_Chart.htm.

11  Katlama, C. *Int. J. Clin. Pract., Suppl.* **1999**, *103*, 16.

12  For reviews on NNRTIs, see: (a) Drake, S. M. *J. Antimicrob. Chemother.* **2000**, *45*, 417; (b) Pedersen, O. S.; Pedersen, E. B. *Synthesis* **2000**, *4*, 479; (c) Hajós, G.; Riedl, Z.; Molnár, J.; Szabó, D. *Drugs of the Future* **2000**, *25*, 47; (d) De Clercq, E. *Antiviral Res.* **1998**, *38*, 153; (e) Sarafianos, S. G.; Das, K.; Ding, J.; Hsiou, Y.; Hughes, S. H.; Arnold, E. In *Anti-Infectives*; Bently, P. H.; O'Hanlon, P. J., Eds.; The Royal Society of Chemistry: Cambridge, 1997, pp. 328–334; (f) Artico, M. *Il Farmaco* **1996**, *51*, 305.

13  For a recent discussion regarding the clinical status of NRTIs and NNRTIs, see: Crowe, S. *Adv. Exp. Med. Biol.* **1999**, *458*, 183.

14  (a) Williams, T. M.; Ciccarone, T. M.; MacTough, S. C.; Rooney, C. S.; Balani, S. K.; Condra, J. H.; Emini, E. A.; Goldman, M. E.; Greenlee, W. J.; Kaufman, L. R.; O'Brien, J. A.; Sardana, V. V.; Schleif, W. A.; Theoharides, A. D.; Anderson, P. S. *J. Med. Chem.* **1993**, *36*, 1291; (b) Young, S. D.; Amblard, M. C.; Britcher, S. F.; Grey, V. E.; Tran, L. O.; Lumma, W. C.; Huff, J. R.; Schleif, W. A.; Emini, E. E.; O'Brien, J. A.; Pettibone, D. J. *Bioorg. Med. Chem. Lett.* **1995**, *5*, 491; (c) Britcher, S. F.; Lumma W. C.; Young, S. D.; Grey, V. E.; Tran, L. O. GB-02282808, 1995.

15  (a) Saari, W. S.; Hoffman, J. M.; Wai, J. S.; Fisher, T. E.; Rooney, C. S.; Smith, A. M.; Thomas, C. M.; Goldman, M. E.; O'Brien, J. A.; Nunberg, J. H.; Quintero, J. C.; Schleif, W. A.; Emini, E. A.; Stern, A. M.; Anderson, P. S. *J. Med. Chem.* **1991**, *34*, 2922; (b) Goldman, M. E.; Nunberg, J. H.; O'Brien, J. A.; Quintero, J. C.; Schleif, W. A.; Freund, K. F.; Gaul, S. L.; Saari, W. S.; Wai, J. S.; Hoffman, J. M.; Anderson, P. S.; Hupe, D. J.; Emini, E. A.; Stern, A. M. *Proc. Natl. Acad. Sci. USA* **1991**, *88*, 6863; (c) Hoffman, J. M.; Wai, J. S.; Thomas,

C. M.; Levin, R. B.; O'Brien, J. A.; Goldman, M. E. *J. Med. Chem.* **1992**, *35*, 3784; (d) Carrol, S. S.; Olsen, D. B.; Bennett, C. D.; Gotlib, L.; Graham, D. J.; Condra, J. H.; Stern, A. M.; Shafer, J. A.; Kuo, L. C. *J. Biol. Chem.* **1993**, *268*, 276; (e) Wai, J. S.; Williams, T. M.; Bamberger, D. L.; Fisher, T. E.; Hoffman, J. M.; Hudcosky, R. J.; MacTough, S. C.; Rooney, C. S.; Saari, W. S.; Thomas, C. M.; Goldman, M. E.; O'Brien, J. A.; Emini, E. A.; Nunberg, J. H.; Quintero, J. C.; Schleif, W. A.; Anderson, P. S. *J. Med. Chem.* **1993**, *36*, 249.

16 Goldman, M. E. In *The Search for Antiviral Drugs – Case Histories from Concept to Clininc*; Adams, J.; Merluzzi, V. J., Eds.; Birkhuser: Boston, 1993, pp. 105–127.

17 Schooley, R. T.; Campbell, T. B.; Kuritzkes, D. R.; Blaschke, T.; Stein, D. S.; Rosandich, M. E.; Phair, J.; Pottage, J. C.; Messari, F.; Collier, A.; Kahn, J. *J. Acquired Immune Deficiency Syndromes Human Retrovirology* **1996**, *12*, 363.

18 Laskin, O. L.; Dupont, A. G.; Buntinx, A.; Schoors, D.; De Pre, M.; Van Hecken, A.; Yeh, K. C.; Woolf, E.; Eisenhandler, R.; De Smet, M.; Patterson, P.; De Lepeleire, I.; De Schepper, P. J. *Antimicrob. Agents Chemother.* **1991**, *31*, 215.

19 Staszewski, S.; Massari, F. E.; Kober, A.; Gohler, R.; Durr, S.; Anderson, K. W.; Schneider, C. L.; Waterbury, J. A.; Bakshi, K. K.; Taylor, V. I.; Hildebrand, C. S.; Kreisl, C.; Hoffstedt, B.; Schleif, W. A.; von Briesen, H.; Rübsamen-Waigmann, H.; Calandra, G. B.; Ryan, J. L.; Stille, W.; Emini, E. A.; Byrnes, V. W. *J. Infectious Diseases* **1995**, *171*, 1159.

20 Davey, R.; Laskin, O.; Decker, M.; O'Neill, D.; Haneiwich, S.; Metcalf, J.; Polis, M.; Kovacs, J.; Davis, S.; Mauer, M.; Yoder, C.; Patterson, P.; Justice, S.; Yeh, K. C.; Woolf, E.; Au, T.; Lane, H. C. *Antimicrob. Agents Chemother.* **1991**, *31*, 215.

21 (a) Tucker, T. J.; Lyle, T. A.; Wiscount, C. M.; Britcher, S. F.; Young, S. D.; Sanders, W. M.; Lumma, W. C.; Goldman, M. E.; O'Brien, J. A.; Ball, R. G.; Homnick, C. F.; Schleif, W. A.; Emini, E. A.; Huff, J. R.; Anderson, P. S. *J. Med. Chem.* **1994**, *37*, 2437; (b) Britcher, S. F.; Lumma, W. C.; Goldman, M. E.; Lyle, T. A.; Huff, J. R.; Payne, L. S.; Quesada, M. L.; Young, S. D.; Sanders, W. M.; Sanderson, P. E.; Tucker, T. J. EP-00530994, 1993.

22 For an alternate preparation of L-738,372, see: Houpis, I. N.; Molina, A.; Douglas, A. W.; Xavier, L.; Lynch, J.; Volante, R. P.; Reider, P. J. *Tetrahedron Lett.* **1994**, *35*, 6811.

23 For enantioselective syntheses of L-738,372, see: (a) Huffman, M. A.; Yasuda, N.; DeCamp, A. E.; Grabowski, E. J. J. *J. Med. Chem.* **1995**, *60*, 1590; (b)Huffman, M. A.; Yasuda, N.; DeCamp, A. E.; Grabowski, E. J. J. WO 9513273, 1995.

24 (a) Britcher, S. F.; Goldman, M. E.; Huff, J. R.; Lumma, W. C.; Lyle, T. A.; Payne, L. S.; Quesda, M. L.; Sanders, W. M.; Sanderson, P. E.; Tucker, T. J.; Young, S. D. WO 9304047, 1992; (b) Britcher, S. F.; Goldman, M. E.; Huff, J. R.; Lumma, W. C.; Lyle, T. A.; Payne, L. S.; Quesda, M. L.; Sanders, W. M.; Sanderson, P. E.; Tucker, T. J.; Young, S. D. EP 530994, 1992; (c) Lyle, T. A.; Tucker, T. J.; Wiscount, C. M. WO 9512583, 1995.

25 (a) Young, S. D.; Britcher, S. F.; Tran, L. O.; Payne, L. S.; Lumma, W. C.; Lyle, T. A.; Huff, J. R.; Anderson, P. S.; Olsen, D. B.; Carrol, S. S.; Pettibone, D. J.; O'Brien, J. A.; Ball, R. G.; Balani, S. K.; Lin, J. H.; Chen, I.; Schleif, W. A.; Sardana, V. V.; Long, W. J.; Byrnes, V. W.; Emini, E. A. *Antimicrob. Agents Chemother.* **1995**, *39*, 2602; (b) Young, S. D.; Britcher, S. F.; Payne, L. S.; Tran, L. O.; Lumma, W. C. US 5,519,021, 1996.

26 Staszewski, S.; Morales-Ramirez, J.; Tashima, K. T.; Rachlis, A.; Skies, D.; Stanford, J.; Stryker, R.; Johnson, P.; Labriola, D. F.; Farina, D.; Manion, D. J.; Ruiz, N. M. *New. Engl. J. Med.* **1999**, *341*, 1865.

27 Bacheler, L.; Weislow, O.; Snyder, S.; Hanna, G.; D'Aquila, R. and the SUSTIVA Resistance Study Team. Abstract presented at the l2th World AIDS Conference, Geneva, Switzerland, June 29–July 3, 1998.

28 (a) Bacheler, L. T. *Drug Resist. Updates* **1999**, *2*, 56–67. (b) Bacheler, L. T.; Cordova, B.; Hanna, G.; D'Aquila, R. D.; Hertogs, K.; Larder, B. Abstract 322. 37th Annual Meeting of the Infectious Deseases Society of America, Philadelphia, PA, November 18–21, 1999. (c) Bacheler, L. T.; Baker, D.; Paul, M.; Jeffrey, S.; Abremski, K. Abstract 2200. 39th Interscience

Conference on Antimicrobial Agents and Chemotherapy, San Francisco, CA, September 26–29, 1999.

29  Hoetelmans, R. M. W. *Antiviral Ther.* **1999**, *4*, 29.

30  Patel, M.; Ko, S. S.; McHugh, R. J., Jr.; Markwalder, J. A.; Srivastava, A. S.; Cordova, B. C.; Klabe, R. M.; Erickson-Viitanen, S.; Trainor, G. L.; Seitz, S. P. *Bioorg. Med. Chem. Lett.* **1999**, *9*, 2805.

31  (a) All compounds were assayed for enzyme activity according to the protocol described in: Sardana, V. V.; Emini, E. A.; Gotlib, L.; Graham, D. J.; Lineberger, D. W.; Long, W. J.; Schlabach, A. J.; Wolfgang, J. A.; Condra, J. H. *J. Biol. Chem.* **1992**, *267*, 17526 using a template primer poly (rA) oligo (dT)$_{12-18}$; (b) All compounds were assayed for whole cell based antiviral activity according to the protocol described in: Bacheler, L. T.; Paul, M.; Jadhav, P. K.; Otto, M.; Miller, J. *Antiviral Chem. Chemother.* **1994**, *5*, 111.

32  The biological activity presented for efavirenz is that of the single enantiomer and, unless reported otherwise, the activity reported for all other compounds is that of the racemate.

33  Patel, M.; McHugh, R. J., Jr.; Cordova, R. M.; Erickson-Viitanen, S.; Trainor, G. L.; Ko, S. S. *Bioorg. Med. Chem. Lett.* **1999**, *9*, 3221.

34  Cocuzza, A. J.; Chidester, D. R.; Cordova, B. C.; Erickson-Viitanen, S.; Trainor, G. L.; Ko, S. S. To be submitted to *Bioorg. Med. Chem. Lett.*

35  Corbett, J. W.; Ko, S. S.; Rodgers, J. D.; Gearhart, L. A.; Magnus, N. A.; Bacheler, L. T.; Diamond, S.; Jeffrey, S.; Klabe, R. M.; Cordova, B. C.; Garber, S.; Logue, K.; Trainor, G. L.; Anderson, P. S.; Erickson-Viitanen, S. K. *J. Med. Chem.* **2000**, *43*, 2019.

36  The racemates contain only 50% of the active enantiomer, and the incorrect enantiomers (the R-isomer) are essentially inactive in the biological assays. Therefore, the activity of the single enantiomers would be expected to be approximately one-half that of the racemic values.

37  Bacheler, L. T. *Drug Resist. Updates* **1999**, *2*, 56–67.

38  Copeland, R. A. *J. Pharm. Sci.* **2000**, *89*, 1000.

39  Corbett, J. W.; Gearhart, L. A.; Ko, S. S.; Rodgers, J. D.; Cordova, B. C.; Klabe, R. M.; Erickson-Viitanen, S. K. *Bioorg. Med. Chem. Lett.* **2000**, *10*, 193.

40  Buckheit, R. W., Jr.; Fliakas-Boltz, V.; Decker, W. D.; Roberson, J. L.; Pyle, C. A.; White, E. L.; Bowdon, B. J.; McMahon, J. B.; Boyd, M. R.; Bader, J. P.; Nickell, D. G.; Barth, H.; Antonucci, T. K. *Antiviral Res.* **1994**, *25*, 43.

41  Wright, J. B. *J. Org. Chem.* **1965**, *30*, 3960

42  Magnus, N. A.; Confalone, P. N.; Storace, L. *Tetrahedron Lett.* **2000**, *41*, 3015.

43  Katritzky, A. R.; Pilarski, B.; Urogdi, L. Synthesis **1989**, 949.

44  Parson, A. F.; Pettifer, R. M. *J. Chem. Soc. Perkin Trans 1* **1998**, *4*, 651.

45  Rodney Parsons of Process Research, DuPont Pharmaceuticals Company, discovered the experimental conditions used to install a PMB-group onto **60**.

46  (a) Kukla, M. J.; Breslin, H. J.; Pauwels, R.; Fedde, C. L.; Miranda, M.; Scott, M. K.; Sherrill, R. G.; Raeymaekers, A.; Van Gelder, J.; Andries, K.; Janssen, M. A. C.; De Clerq, E. D.; Janssen, P. A. *J. Med. Chem.* **1991**, *34*, 746; (b) Kukla, M. J.; Breslin, H. J.; Diamond, C. J.; Grous, P. P.; Ho, C. Y.; Miranda, Milton; Rodgers, M. J.; Sherrill, R. G.; De Clercq, E.; Pauwels, R.; Andries, K.; Moens, L. J.; Janssen, M. A. C.; Janssen, P. A. J. *J. Med. Chem.* **1991**, *34*, 3187.

47  (a) Bell, F. W.; Cantrell, A. S.; Hoegberg, M.; Jaskunas, S. R.; Johansson, N. G.; Jordan, C. L.; Kinnick, M. D.; Lind, P.; Morin, J. M., Jr.; Noréen, R.; Öberg, B.; Palkowitz, J. A.; Parrish, C. A.; Pranc, P.; Sahlberg, C.; Ternansky, R. J.; Vasileff, R. T.; Vrang, L.; West, S. J.; Zhang, H.; Zhou, X.-X. *J. Med. Chem.* **1995**, 38, 4929. (b) Cantrell, A. S.; Engelhardt, P.; Hoegberg, M.; Jaskunas, S. R.; Johansson, N. G.; Jordan, C. L.; Kangasmetsae, J.; Kinnick, M. D.; Lind, P.; Morin, J. M., Jr.; Muesing, M. A.; Noreén, R.; Öberg, B.; Pranc, P.; Sahlberg, C.; Ternansky, R. J.; Vasileff, R. T.; Vrang, L.; West, S. J.; Zhang H. *J. Med. Chem.* **1996**, *39*, 4261.

48  Mike, W. et al. 6th Conference on Retrovirus and Opportunistic Infections.

49  Ring, N.; Nusrat, R.; Lazzarin, A.; Arasteh, K.; Goebel, F.P.; Audagnotto, S.; Rachlis, A.; Arribas, J.R.; Ploughman, L.; Fiske, W.; Labriola, D.; Levy, R.; Echols, R., 9th Conference on Retrovirus and Opportunistic Infections; February 24–28, 2002.

Progress in Medicinal Chemistry – Vol. 40,
Series Editors: F.D. King and A.W. Oxford
Guest Editors: A.B. Reitz and S.L. Dax

# 4 Molecular Modeling of Opioid Receptor-Ligand Complexes

IAIN McFADYEN, THOMAS METZGER,
GOVINDAN SUBRAMANIAN, GENNADY PODA,
ERIK JORVIG AND DAVID M. FERGUSON*

*Department of Medicinal Chemistry,
University of Minnesota, Minneapolis, MN 55455*

INTRODUCTION

Opioid receptors mediate the effects of a wide array of endogenous peptides and exogenous alkaloids, including clinically useful analgesics such as morphine [1]. Upon activation, opioid receptors couple *via* intracellular heterotrimeric G proteins to influence a number of signaling pathways. Specifically, selective interaction with members of the $G_i$ and $G_o$ families leads to inhibition of adenylyl cyclase, activation of inwardly rectifying potassium channels, and inhibition of voltage dependent calcium channels [2–5]. The resulting physiological effects are diverse, and include analgesia, euphoria, respiratory depression, inhibition of gastrointestinal mobility, nausea, and development of tolerance and dependence [6].

Decades of structure-activity relationship research seeking to divorce the potent analgesia of opioids from this plethora of undesirable side effects has produced a staggering diversity of compounds [7,8]. The most numerous and best characterized class of opioid ligands is termed the 'opiates,' comprising those compounds which share the characteristic fused ring 'morphinan' skeleton [8]. Perhaps unsurprisingly, the search for the 'perfect' analgesic has met with limited success–morphine remains the analgesic agent of choice in cases of severe chronic pain [9]. However, these synthetic efforts have provided researchers with a comprehensive array of pharmacological tools covering the spectrum of structure, affinity, efficacy and selectivity [1].

The existence of opioid receptors types was initially proposed in the 1970's based on the pharmacological characterization of certain prototypical opiates [10]. The evidence for types mounted in the years following, culminating in the cloning of the mu, delta and kappa receptors in the early 1990's (see references [11–14]. for reviews). Sequence analysis suggests that the cloned opioid receptors are members of the superfamily of G protein-coupled receptors (GPCRs), as has been confirmed by a variety of experimental evidence. Thus, they are characterized by seven alpha helical transmembrane (TM) domains connected by three intracellular and three extracellular loops. The extracellular (EL) N-terminus and the intracellular (IL) C-terminus are both targets for post-translational glycosylation. For a serpentine representation of this structure, see *Figure 4.1*.

As noted by Baldwin *et al.*, [15] GPCRs contain a characteristic set of residues largely located within the transmembrane domains which are highly or even absolutely conserved across the entire family. The mu, delta, and kappa opioid receptors contain almost all of these residues. Within the opioid receptor family, the three types share approximately 60% sequence identity, rising to 70% in the transmembrane domain. The most variable regions include the termini and extracellular loops 2 and 3. Mu, delta and kappa receptors have since been cloned from a variety of mammalian species, and in each case

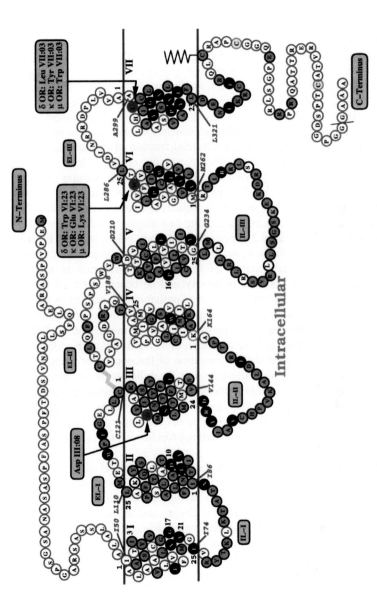

*Figure 4.1. Serpentine model of the delta opioid receptor showing the transmembrane (TM), loop, and N/C terminal domains. Residues conserved within the ORD, ORK, and ORM are shown in grey. The highly conserved residues (>90%) across all aminergic receptors are black. Amino acid residues are numbered according to their relative position in each domain. For example, the conserved Asp in TM III is referred to as Asp III:08, indicating the 8th position from the N-terminal end of the helix. Key residues involved in ligand binding are shown in red.*

sequence identity between homologs is greater than 90%. There is evidence that opioid receptors have been present throughout vertebrate and even invertebrate evolution [16–21]. A schematic of the delta opioid receptor is given in Figure 4.1.

In the quest to understand the relationship between structure and function in the opioid receptors, a wide variety of biophysical and molecular biological techniques have been applied. These include the creation of single or multiple point mutants, chimeric receptors, and metal ion binding sites, the substituted cysteine accessibility method (SCAM), use of fluorescent or spin labels, and more. By far the most popular of these approaches has been single point mutagenesis [22]. Indeed, mutants at a substantial fraction of the residues in the putative transmembrane domains of the three opioid receptors have been reported (see for example http://www.opioid.umn.edu), with the aim of elucidating their role(s) in ligand binding and/or receptor activation.

However, it is vital that data from such mutants not be over-interpreted. The effect(s) of a certain mutation on the binding of a single ligand or a subset of ligands cannot be extrapolated to apply to all ligands belonging to a broader class. For example, a decrease in the binding affinity of DAMGO (a mu-selective peptide) to a certain mutant of the mu opioid receptor in no way guarantees that a similar decrease in affinity will be observed for all mu-selective ligands, agonists, or even peptides. Similarly, the fact that a certain mutation causes a significant change in ligand binding characteristics does not necessarily imply that the residue in question interacts directly with the ligand. Other possible explanations include alteration of accessibility to the pocket, an indirect (allosteric) action on the conformation of the pocket, or even a generalized change in the overall conformation or flexibility of the receptor. Thus data from 'gain of function' or reciprocal mutants is preferable, although unfortunately much less common, than that from 'loss of function' mutagenesis experiments [23]. Nevertheless, when interpreted cautiously the wealth of data which is available from these experimental approaches is of great utility to the molecular modeler.

Molecular models of GPCRs can be used at a number of different levels, from visualization to complex theoretical simulations. A common use of such models is in conjunction with molecular biological approaches in a cyclical progression of visualization, experimental design, and model refinement [24]. For others, models provide a key tool with which to investigate the relationship between structure and function at the molecular level, for example the mechanisms underlying ligand binding, selectivity and activation. Finally, molecular models form an integral part of any rational drug design strategy, through docking studies, database screening, *de novo* ligand design and so forth [25]. In the case of the opioid receptors, molecular modeling approaches have the potential to increase our understanding of ligand-receptor interactions enormously, and thereby provide the breakthrough in analgesic drug design which has so far proved elusive. Obviously, the reliability and usefulness of the results from all molecular modeling studies are limited by the accuracy of the model itself. Ideally, models would be constructed directly from high-resolution experimental structures; of course, this is rarely possible since the number of cloned sequences vastly outweighs the number of available structures [26,27]. For example, the curated database SWISS-PROT[28] (ca.expasy.org/sprot/) contained 93,435 non-redundant sequences as of release 39.14, dated 21st February 2001, compared with 10,833 possibly redundant x-ray structures of varying resolution in the 20th February 2001 update of the Research Collaboratory for Structural Bioinformatics Protein Database, previously the Brookhaven PDB (www.rcsb.org/pdb/) [29].

In the absence of experimental structures of the target protein itself, model building is typically achieved through homology or heuristic-based modeling. Here the sequence of the target protein is 'threaded' onto a 'template', a known high-resolution structure of a (preferably closely) related protein, based upon a sequence alignment [27,30]. The implicit assumption is that the template is likely to be similar enough in structure to the target that the end result is a reliable model. The relationship between sequence identity and structural similarity is well known [26,31], but the key question regards the cut-off in sequence identity below which reasonable structural similarity is lost and homology modeling techniques become unreliable. This varies largely as a function of the ease of construction of an unambiguous sequence alignment [30,32].

Although over a thousand GPCRs have now been cloned, they are amongst the most difficult of all proteins to purify and crystallize due to problems of solubility and lability. Therefore until very recently, all attempts to solve their structure at atomic resolution have been unsuccessful. In the absence of a high-resolution template suitable for homology modeling, extensive efforts has been devoted to modeling GPCRs using alternative strategies. Here we review the various methodologies which have been applied in modeling the opioid receptors, and the results of our own model building efforts. We also present the results of docking studies using certain prototypical opioid ligands, which when combined with available mutagenesis and pharmacological data allow us to propose a structure-based rationale for their type selectivity (or lack thereof).

## HISTORICAL PERSPECTIVE

Regardless of the strategy used in modeling a GPCR, the key first step is to define the extents of the α-helices that are to be modeled. This is typically achieved through analysis of one or more physical characteristics of the receptor sequence or, more commonly, of a multiple sequence alignment of related receptors. For example, the majority of residues within the transmembrane domains are in contact with either the lipid bilayer or other helices and are therefore likely to be more hydrophobic than residues in the intra- or extracellular domains exposed to an aqueous environment. Thus, a plot of the rolling average hydrophobicity along the sequence may reveal those segments of the sequence which are buried in the membrane [33].

The α-helices may extend beyond the boundaries of the lipid portion of the membrane where the residues necessarily are predominantly hydrophobic, into the charged head groups or even beyond [34]. More sophisticated approaches take advantage of the fact that α-helices typically show periodicity in several properties, including hydrophobicity, conservation and substitution patterns [35]. For example, those residues with important functional or structural roles are likely to be more conserved than would be expected. These presumably face the interior of the receptor or other helices rather than the lipid. Analysis using Fourier transform methods can reveal this periodicity, and thereby help to locate and define helical segments [35]. Further, statistical methods have shown that certain residues appear more or less frequently than would be expected in helices or in characteristic helix capping motifs [36–38].

It must be emphasized that all such approaches carry inherent limitations and yield predictions for helix boundaries which may be in error by as much as 2 helical turns (up to 7 or 8 residues) [25]. For example, periodicity analysis assumes the presence of ideal α-helices, that are straight, regular, vertical, and amphiphilic in character [39]. Obviously this is unlikely to hold true for real-world membrane proteins, as has been shown for both bacteriorhodopsin and rhodopsin [40,41]. Furthermore, estimates from different analyses typically yield conflicting predictions for helix boundaries. A common approach is to apply two or more analyses and take a consensus between the various predictions [34]. Although this is obviously not an ideal situation, as long as care is taken to include all residues implicated in ligand binding or structural roles then the exact definition of helix boundaries is not critical. For an extensive review of the techniques which can be applied to predicting helical boundaries and the problems associated with them, see Ballesteros and Weinstein [34].

## BACTERIORHODOPSIN BASED MODELS

Many early GPCR modeling efforts used the structure of the bacterial light sensing protein bacteriorhodopsin as a template (at that time the only 7TM receptor whose structure had been solved at high resolution) [42,43]. This approach involves the dual implicit assumptions that bacteriorhodopsin shares a common overall fold with the GPCRs and that a meaningful sequence alignment can be constructed between them. However, although bacteriorhodopsin shares the seven alpha-helical transmembrane domains characteristic of GPCRs, it does not couple to a G protein, instead acting as a proton pump [42]. Such a marked difference in function likely corresponds with significant differences in three-dimensional structure. Indeed, comparison of the structures of bacteriorhodopsin and the G protein-coupled receptor rhodopsin reveals striking differences in helix positions, tilts and kinks [39]. Furthermore, bacteriorhodopsin shares little sequence homology with any known GPCR (<15%). Thus, in the absence of many of the conserved residues found throughout the GPCR family, the construction of a meaningful sequence alignment is far from trivial. Taken together, these concerns make the use of bacteriorhodopsin as a template for homology modeling of GPCRs highly questionable, and this approach has largely fallen out of favor.

## DE NOVO APPROACHES

In cases where no reliable template exists for homology modeling, one alternative is to construct a model *de novo*. This approach has been applied in several instances to GPCRs, and although the details vary, there is a common overall procedure. Idealized helices are built with standard right-handed $\alpha$-helical backbone torsion angles ($\phi = -65°$, $\psi = -40°$), with or without proline kink parameters. The same Fourier transform procedures described above can be used to analyze property profiles such as hydrophobicity, conservation, or solvent accessibility and thereby provide estimates as to the interior face of the various helices [35,44]. Similarly, the extent of exposure of the helix to lipid serves to orient the helices with respect to one another [15,45]. This information is used to assemble the helices into a bundle which is then subjected to energy minimization and/or molecular dynamics. However, this approach suffers from several obvious limitations, not the least of which is difficulty in dealing with helix tilts (see for example [46]).

## RHODOPSIN BASED MODELS

The most widely accepted approach to modeling GPCRs in recent years involves the use of rhodopsin as a partial structural 'template'. Rhodopsin is structurally related to bacteriorhodopsin in that both are 7TM light sensing proteins with a covalently attached ligand, namely retinal [39]. However, rhodopsin is much more suitable as a template for GPCR modeling than bacteriorhodopsin. Rhodopsin couples to the G protein transducin, and all members of the GPCR superfamily presumably share a common overall three dimensional structure, at least in the transmembrane regions, due to the necessary conservation of signal transduction functions. Although sequence identity with other GPCRs is quite low within the transmembrane domains, about 23–25% in the case of the opioid receptors, rhodopsin contains most of the highly conserved residues characteristic of GPCRs [15]. This greatly facilitates the construction of multiple sequence alignments and thus makes homology modeling a feasible proposition.

Rhodopsin is available natively in abundant quantity and relatively high concentration in the outer segments of retinal rod cells [47], and is therefore a natural target for attempts to crystallize a GPCR. Nevertheless, despite much effort from many laboratories, three dimensional crystals suitable for x-ray diffraction studies were not obtained until very recently. However, two dimensional rhodopsin crystals from a variety of species have given low resolution projection structures *via* electron cryo-microscopy [39]. In a seminal early contribution, Baldwin *et al.* [45] deduced the probable common arrangement of the helices and assigned them to the density contours seen in the earliest 9 Å structure of bovine rhodopsin [48] by analyzing the structural information contained in a multiple sequence alignment of over 200 GPCRs. The model was later updated to include many more GPCR sequences and newly available higher resolution rhodopsin structures (5–6 Å, for review see [39]). The resulting α-carbon only 'structure' of rhodopsin remained until very recently the best template for GPCR modeling efforts. However, since the template itself is of less than atomic resolution there is some uncertainty as to the accuracy of the models derived from it. Although this is difficult to assess independently, it is generally acknowledged that the relative depth and orientation of the helices are accurate only to within 1–2 vertical turns and as much as 100° rotation, respectively [25]. Therefore great care must be taken not to over-interpret results gained from studies on such models.

Perhaps the most exciting developments in the use of rhodopsin-based templates has been the determination of atomic resolution crystal coordinates for rhodopsin [41,49]. At 2.1 angstroms, a vast array of structural details are evident, including pi-bulges, $3_{10}$ helical segments, and numerous hydrogen bonding networks within the TM helices. While this data has shed new insight to the structural basis to the molecular conformation and function of rhodopsin, the sparse sequence identity shared with the opioid family (as well as other aminergic GPCRs) limits the use of this information in model building. (A detailed accounting the molecular conformation of rhodopsin is given in references [41] and [49].)

Even within rhodopsin-based model building procedures, there is wide variation in the subsequent stages of model refinement, arising from the type and number of distance constraints used. A typical approach involves incorporating distance constraints gained from mutagenesis and other protein engineering studies. Alternatively, the model can be refined using only simulated helical backbone hydrogen bond constraints, and the experimentally derived distance constraints can then be used later to validate the model. In a novel approach, Pogozheva *et al.* have built GPCR models using an iterative refinement procedure aiming to saturate the hydrogen bonding potential gleaned from an ensemble of receptors, based upon the interactions between polar residues on different helices [50,51].

## LIGAND-RECEPTOR COMPLEXES

One of the most popular applications of molecular models of GPCRs is in docking studies. An emerging technique which has gained a large following in the pharmaceutical industry is the 'virtual screening' of large (potentially massive) compound libraries aiming to identify potential 'lead' compounds [52]. However, in the opioid field docking studies have typically been performed with relatively small sets of structurally rigid opiates in order to probe the mechanisms of ligand binding or to validate molecular models [53].

The docking of ligands to a receptor model is a two step process. In the first stage, the various ligands are docked into the active site of the receptor, and multiple plausible orientations are reported. A number of docking programs utilizing a variety of different algorithms are available, with one of the key distinctions between the various methods being their treatment of the conformational flexibility of the ligand(s). Although ideally the docking program would also take into account conformational freedom of the receptor, in the majority of cases this is currently not feasible due to time constraints and limitations in computational power. The second stage involves scoring the docked ligands for the 'goodness' or complementarity of their fit to the receptor, and reporting a ranked list. Again, a wide variety of programs are available, and several reviews have focused on the relative performance of different combinations of docking and scoring functions in different situations (for example, see [54,55]). Regardless of the program(s) used, accurate and reliable prediction of the affinity of ligands for receptors remains a difficult task. However, there have been many successful applications of docking studies to library screening, mechanistic studies and model validation.

## MODELING METHODOLOGY

### GENERAL METHODS/PROTOCOLS

Helix building was accomplished using the Insight II package from Biosym, and MidasPlus was used throughout for visualization [56,57]. All energy minimization and molecular dynamics were performed *in vacuo* using the AMBER 5.0 suite of programs [58] with the Cornell *et al.* all-atom force field,

[59] a non-bonded cut-off distance of 8.0 Å and a distance-dependant dielectric of 4*r*. The DOCK 3.5 suite of programs was used to perform the docking procedures [60,61]. In the SPHGEN module, limits of 2.3 Å and 2.8 Å were assigned to polar and hydrophobic contacts respectively, while 'good contacts' were limited to 4.5 Å.

## RECEPTOR MODEL BUILDING

The sequences for the rat mu, mouse delta, and rat kappa opioid receptors were retrieved from the SWISS-PROT [28] online database (accession numbers P33535, P32300, and P34975 respectively). In order to find all GPCRs sharing >30% homology with the opioid receptors, similarity searching was performed across multiple databases using BlastP [62]. A total of 56 non-redundant sequences were retrieved, of which a multiple sequence alignment was created using ClustalW [63]. All highly conserved residues were correctly aligned in all sequences [15].

Residues are referred to throughout by their position in the primary sequence (e.g. Trp304) and also by the generic GPCR numbering scheme whereby roman numerals indicate TM helix and arabic numerals denote position from the N-terminal end of that helix [15]. For example Leu300 in delta, Trp320 in mu, and Tyr312 in kappa all occupy the same relative position in the seventh trans-membrane region and are therefore all referred to as VII:03. (See *Figure 4.1* for additional information.)

The helix boundaries were predicted from the multiple sequence alignment using the PHDhtm module of PredictProtein [64], and refined based upon analyis of N- and C-terminal helix capping motifs [65]. The consensus helix extents are shown in a sequence alignment of the mu, delta and kappa opioid receptors given in *Figure 4.2*. All predicted transmembrane domains were free of gaps. Helices I through VI were modeled as idealized right-handed α-helices, using standard backbone torsion angles ($\phi = -65°$, $\psi = -40°$). Averaged proline kink angles [66] were introduced in TMs V and VI (Pro V: 16 and Pro VI: 15), as seen in the Baldwin model of rhodopsin [15]. Analyses of available experimental evidence required that special consideration be given to modeling TM VII. A unique pattern of spatial contacts between TM VII and three other helices, TMs I, II, and III, (I: 18-II: 10-VII: 17; II: 10-III:04-VII: 11 [67,68,69], are not easily accommodated using an ideal α-helical conformation for TM VII. In addition, accessibility profiles of TM VII of the dopamine $D_2$-receptor determined using sulfhydryl-specific reagents are inconsistent with an α-helical conformation of this TM domain [70]. To account for these observations, we have modeled TM VII as a piece of $33_{10}$-helix (from Gly VII: 10 to Pro VII: 18), flanked on both sides by α-helical segments. All helices were subsequently

**N-Terminus**

```
Delta   1  MELVP-----S------ARAELQSSP--LVNLSDAFPSAFPSACANASGSPG------ARSASSLALA  49
Mu      1  MDSSTGPGNTSDCSDPLAQASCSPAPGSWLNLSHVDGNQSDPCSLNRTGLGCNDSLCPQTSSPSMVTA  68
Kappa   1  MESPIQIFRGE------PGPTCAPSACLLPNSSSWFPNWAESDSNGSVGSEDQQ---LEPAHISPAIP  59
           *:              .   .:.      * *      .     *      .     *   *
```

**Helix 1**                1                    29              **Intracellular Loop 1**
```
Delta   50  IAITALYSAVCAVGLLGNVLVMFGIVR  76      77  YTKL  80
Mu      69  ITIMALYSIVCVVGLFGNFLVMYVIVR  95      96  YTKM  99
Kappa   60  VIITAVYSVVFVVGLVGNSLVMFVIIR  86      87  YTKM  90
            ; * *;** * .***.** ***; *;*          ***;
```

**Helix 2**                0                    29              **Extracellular Loop 1**
```
Delta   81  KTATNIYIFNLALADALATSTLPFQSAKYL  110    111  METWPFGELL  120
Mu     100  KTATNIYIFNLALADALATSTLPFQSVNYL  129    130  MGTWPFGTIL  139
Kappa   91  KTATNIYIFNLALADALVTTTMPFQSAVYL  120    121  MNSWPFGDVL  130
            ***************** .*:*:**** **       * ;**** ;*
```

**Helix 3**                0                     32             **Intracellular Loop 2**
```
Delta  121  CKAVLSIDYYNMFTSIFTLTMMSVDRYIAVCHP  153    154  VKALDFRT  161
Mu     140  CKIVISIDYYNMFTSIFTLCTMSVDRYIAVCHP  172    173  VKALDFRT  180
Kappa  131  CKIVISIDYYNMFTSIFTLTMMSVDRYIAVCHP  163    164  VKALDFRT  171
            ** *;*************** ************          ********
```

**Helix 4**                0                25                 **Extracellular Loop 2**
```
Delta  162  PAKAKLINICIWVLASGVGVPIMVMA  187    188  VTQPRDGA--VVCMLQFPSPSW-YW  209
Mu     181  PRNAKIVNVCNWILSSAIGLPVMFMA  206    207  TTKYRQGS--IDCTLTFSHPTW-YW  228
Kappa  172  PLKAKIINICIWLLASSVGISAIVLG  197    198  GTKVREDVDVIECSLQFPDDEYSWW  222
            * ;**;;*;* *;*;*.;*;. ;.:.       *; *;.    ; * * *.   ;;*
```

**Helix 5**                -1                   30             **Intracellular Loop 3**
```
Delta  210  DTVTKICVFLFAFVVPILIITVCYGLMLLRLR  241    242  SVRLLSGSKEKDRSLR  257
Mu     229  ENLLKICVFIFAFIMPVLIITVCYGLMILRLK  260    261  SVRMLSGSKEKDRNLR  276
Kappa  223  DLFMKICVFVPAFVIPVLIIIVCYTLMILRLK  254    255  SVRLLSGSREKDRNLR  270
            ; . *****;***;;*;*** *** **;***;        ***;****;****.**
```

**Helix 6**                0                   28              **Extracellular Loop 3**
```
Delta  258  RITRMVLVVVGAFVVCWAPIHIFVIVWTL  286    287  VDINRRDPLVVA  298
Mu     277  RITRMVLVVVAVFIVCWTPIHIYVIIKAL  305    306  ITIP-ETFFQTV  316
Kappa  271  RITKLVLVVVAVFIICWTPIHIFILVEAL  299    300  GSTS-HSTAVLS  310
            ***;;*****.*.*;;**;****;;;; ;*
```

**Helix 7**                2                   29
```
Delta  299  ALHLCIALGYANSSLNPVLYAFLDENFK  326
Mu     317  SWHFCIALGYTNSCLNPVLYAFLDENFK  344
Kappa  311  SYYFCIALGYTNSSLNPVLYAFLDENFK  338
            : ;;******;** .**************
```

**C-Terminus**
```
Delta  327  RCFRQLCRTPCGRQEPGSLRRPRQATTRERVTACTPS------DGPGGGAAA--  372
Mu     345  RCFREFCIPTSSTIEQQNSTRVRQNTREHPSTANTVDRTNHQLENLEAETAPLP  398
Kappa  339  RCFRDFCFPIKMRMERQSTNRVR-NTVQDPASMRDVG---------GMNKPV-  380
            ****;;*  .    *  .; * * *    .          :
```

*Figure 4.2.    Alignment of the sequences of the mu, kappa, and delta opioid receptors. The sequences used are all from SWISS-PROT (ID, accession number): mu (OPRM_RAT, P33535); delta (OPRD_MOUSE, P32300); kappa (0PRK_RAT, P34975). Consensus key: * - fully conserved residue, : - strong conservation,. - weak conservation (as defined by Clustal W).*

capped with acetyl (ACE) and N-methyl (NME) groups at the N- and C-terminus, respectively. The modeled helices were threaded onto the rhodopsin template of Baldwin *et al.* through superimposition of the common $C_\alpha$ atoms [15]. The relative rotation and depth of the various helices were manually examined to assess compatibility with the available data from substitutedcysteine accessibility method (SCAM) and mutagenesis experiments [15,70–72]. Initial side chain torsional angles were generated using SCWRL [73], which uses a backbone-dependent rotamer library [74]. In each case a small number of sidechain-sidechain clashes were unresolved by SCWRL and were manually adjusted prior to model refinement.

MODEL REFINEMENT

In order to fully relax side chain packing, the starting structures of the helical bundles for the mu, delta, and kappa receptors were subjected to energy minimization with strong positional constraints on all backbone atoms (5 $kcal/\mathring{A}^2/mol$) until the RMS deviation of the gradient reached $0.001\,kcal/mol/\mathring{A}$. The first 100 steps of this minimization used the steepest descent method, with the remainder following the conjugate gradient method. This was followed by 400ps of molecular dynamics (MD) simulation using a step size of 1 fs under constant temperature conditions at 300K. Backbone constraints designed to simulate $C=O_i\ldots H-N_{i+4}$ hydrogen bonds were gradually reduced from $5\,kcal/\mathring{A}^2/mol$ to $0.05\,kcal/\mathring{A}^2/mol$ over the course of the first 300ps of the MD run, and then maintained at $0.05\,kcal/\mathring{A}/mol$ for the last 100ps. The averaged receptor structure from the last 50ps of the trajectory was subjected to a final energy minimization with reduced positional constraints on backbone atoms ($2\,kcal/\mathring{A}^2/mol$).

The overall structural quality of the models was assessed using PROCHECK [75], which showed that in each case >96% of the residues were in the most favorable region of the Ramachandran plot whilst the remaining residues were in the additionally allowed region. Likewise, side chain dihedral angles were in the most favorable regions for >97% residues and the remainder were in the additionally allowed regions. There were no bad side chain contacts in any of the models. The RMS deviations of the models from the Baldwin *et al.* rhodopsin template [15] were 1.81 Å for delta, 1.78 Å for mu, and 1.75 Å for kappa when considering shared $C_\alpha$ atoms only.

LIGAND DOCKING

The names and structures of the ligands used in the docking studies are shown in *Figure 4.3*. The starting structures were taken from the relevant crystal

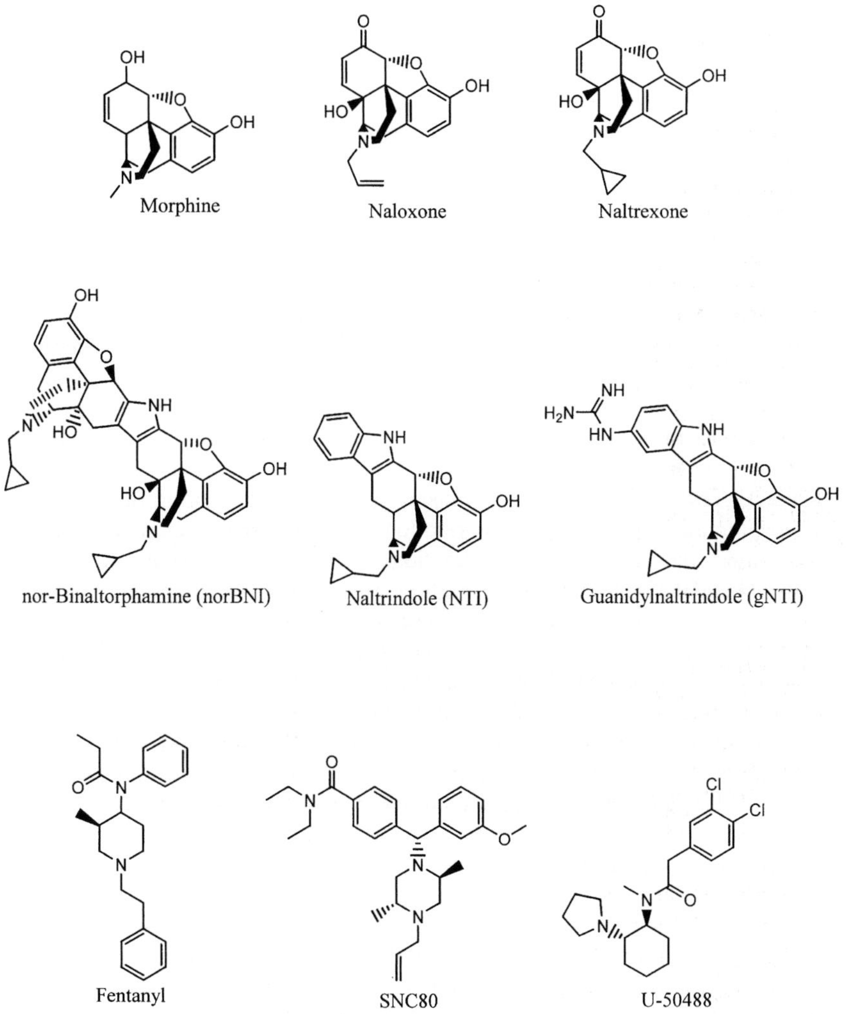

Figure 4.3. Opioid ligands.

structures deposited in the Cambridge Structural Database, maintained by the Cambridge Crystallographic Data Center (http://www.ccdc.cam.ac.uk/) where possible. The remaining ligand starting structures were model built from closely related X-ray structures using Insight II. All ligands were considered in their biologically relevant protonated species. The starting geometries of the ligands were subjected to *ab initio* energy minimization at the HF/6-31G* level using the Gaussian98 package [76]. The restrained electrostatic potential (RESP) charge fitting formalism was employed to derive partial atomic charges [77]. In order to maintain consistency, the ligands were then subjected to the same minimization procedure as the receptor models, described above. Additional bond lengths, bond angles, dihedrals, and improper torsion angles not found in the parm94.dat force field were derived by analogy and from explicit parameterization of the torsional profiles of smaller ligand fragments.

A solvent accessible molecular surface of the receptor (SAMS) was generated using the Connelly algorithm [78], and the program SPHGEN was used to fill the cavities on the interior of this surface. As noted elsewhere [79], this procedure tends to produce an overly large set of spheres which must be examined and trimmed manually. In each case the final sphere set consisted of 40–80 spheres which serve to define the extents of the putative ligand binding pocket.

A number of docking orientations were generated for each ligand using the SINGLE module of DOCK, allowing a maximum of two to six bad steric contacts. These orientations were ranked by a force-field scoring function ($E_{ff}$) which summed the empirical contributions from electrostatics, van der Waals repulsions, and van der Waals attractions, as measured using the DISTMAP and CHEMGRID modules. The highest ranking docked alignments of each ligand were manually examined to assess their agreement with mutagenesis data. Specifically, the most widely recognized and best characterized point of interaction between opioid ligands and their receptors is between the protonated nitrogen and the side chain of an aspartate residue in TM III (III:08, Asp128 in delta, Asp147 in mu, Asp138 in kappa) respectively, presumably through the formation of a salt bridge [22]. In some cases, docking orientations which fulfilled this requirement were scored lower than those which did not. Close examination of the scoring results showed that this was primarily due to an over-emphasis in the unrefined ligand-receptor complex on van der Waals repulsions between the ligands and side chains which could be relieved by subsequent minimization and/or molecular dynamics. For these ligands the lower scoring arrangements which fulfilled the cationic amine to aspartate (III:08) salt bridge requirement were selected. A complete discussion of this problem in the automated docking of fentanyl compounds to the mu-opioid receptor has been reported by us [80].

In order to relieve any unfavorable steric interactions, the starting ligand-receptor complexes were subjected to energy minimization and molecular dynamics, following the protocols outlined above for the receptor models. Briefly, an initial energy minimization with strong (5 kcal/Å/mol) positional constraints on receptor backbone atoms was followed by 400ps of MD simulations. The averaged ligand-receptor structure from the last 50ps of the trajectory was subjected to a final energy minimization, as above.

## RESULTS AND DISCUSSION

### TM DOMAIN

Approximately 70% (137 of 205) residues in the transmembrane domains, as defined in this study, are conserved across the mu, delta, and kappa opioid receptor types. Of the seven helices, the most conserved are TMs II, III, and VII, while the least conserved is TM IV. In general, the central and intracellular portions of the bundle are the most conserved, while the extracellular ends of the helices appear more variable. Within the conserved regions are several extensive networks of hydrogen bonds and aromatic-aromatic interactions, which have been described in detail previously. These interactions have been proposed to play roles both in maintaining receptor structure and in receptor activation.

As identified by DOCK, the binding pocket is very similar in each of the mu, delta and kappa types, and is situated between TMs III, V, VI and VII. The sphere cluster generated by DOCK is shown in *Figure 4.4*. The pocket extends from the extracellular surface to approximately one third to one quarter of the depth of the helical bundle. The environment surrounding the binding pocket mirrors the general pattern of conservation seen in the transmembrane bundle as a whole. Thus, there is a gradual shift from residues that are highly conserved throughout the GPCR family at the deepest end of the pocket, to residues invariant in the opioid receptor family at the mid-point of the pocket, to highly variable residues at the extracellular interface. There are only two residues in the vicinity of the binding pocket which are type specific, i.e. unique in each of the mu, delta and kappa receptors, namely VI:23 (Trp284 in delta, Lys303 in mu, Glu297 in kappa) and VII:03 (Leu300 in delta, Trp318 in mu, Tyr312 in kappa).

### DOCKING RESULTS

It is useful to consider the results from the docking studies in terms of the 'message-address' concept of Portoghese [81], which seeks to rationalize the type selectivity of opioid ligands. The theory states that opioid ligands contain three distinct moieties. The 'message' moiety is common to all ligands, is typically considered to be the tyramine group containing the cationic amine. The 'address' moiety varies from ligand to ligand and is connected to the 'message' via a spacer, whose only role is to correctly orient the functional parts of the ligand. Likewise, the ligand binding pocket in opioid receptors comprises two spatially overlapping yet functionally distinct recognition sites. The first confers high affinity binding by accommodating the 'message' moiety, with a binding arrangement which is proposed to be largely similar in each of the mu,

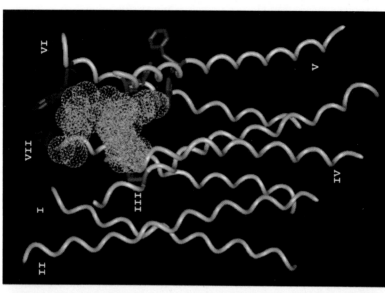

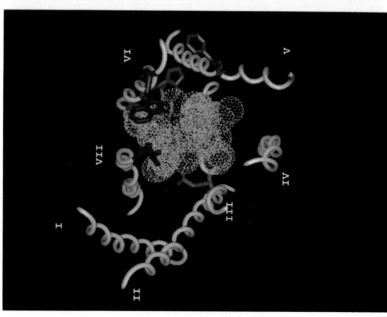

*Figure 4.4.   Orthogonal views of DOCK generated sphere cluster used in automated docking to the delta opioid receptor. The spheres (yellow) fill the binding cavity encompassed by the conserved Asp in TM III (III:08 in red), a cluster of aromatic residues in TM V and VI (Phe V: 13, Trp VI: 14, and His VI: 17 in green), and a putative selectivity site at the TM VI-VII (Trp VI:03 and Leu VII:03 blue). The TM helices are numbered in white. This*

delta and kappa receptors. As a corollary, this area of the pocket must itself be conserved throughout the opioid receptor family. A second recognition site is responsible for conferring type selectivity through specific interactions with the 'address', either by increasing the affinity of favored ligands, decreasing the affinity of non-favored ligands, or both. The 'address' recognition site must therefore be variable between the three opioid receptor types.

## NALOXONE AND RELATED OPIATES

The results of docking the non-selective antagonist naloxone are similar for all three opioid receptor types. In all cases, the relatively small naloxone occupies only the deepest portion of the binding pocket in the region spanning TMs III, VI, and VII (as shown in *Figure 4.5*). The majority of the residues in close proximity to the ligand are conserved across the opioid receptor family, while the remainder are relatively conservative mutations such as to Val or to Leu. The cationic amine of naloxone is involved in a salt bridge interaction with Asp III:08, while the aromatic ring is surround by Tyr III:09, His VI: 17, and other, mostly aromatic, residues. Similar results are obtained with other non-selective opiate ligands including naltrexone, diprenorphine, bremazocine and ethylketazocine (results not shown). These non-selective ligands can be thought of as comprising the opioid 'message' with no 'address' moiety. Thus, the observed similarities in the binding modes of these ligands to the mu, delta and kappa types and the high degree of conservation in the surrounding residues are in close agreement with the 'message-address' concept. In addition, the docking mode for these 'message' type compounds as established by DOCK is in agreement with the mode determined by *de novo* methods based on ligand structure, site-directed mutagenesis results and other model building and ligand structure-activity heuristics [53].

Over the years, a number of selective opioid ligands have been directly derived from the naltrexone scaffold including the kappa-selective antagonists norbinaltorphamine (norBNI) and guanidinylnaltrindole (GNTI) and the delta-selective antagonist naltrindole (NTI). An alignment of the universal message displayed by these ligands can be applied to explore the 'address' site(s) within the opioid receptors. The resulting binding site model locates the naltrexone core or opioid message in the conserved binding pocket within the TM domain (equivalent to that of naloxone shown in *Figure 4.5*) with the selective or 'address' portions of the ligand projected towards the upper boundary of the TM-extracellular loop boundary region between TM helices VI and VII [53]. The docked structure of GNTI is given in *Figure 4.6*. In this binding orientation, the ligand address components (the indole moiety for delta and the positively charged nitrogen for kappa) are directed towards environments or pockets in the receptor that are type specific. In terms of unique residues or sites

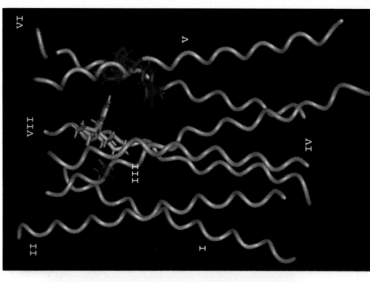

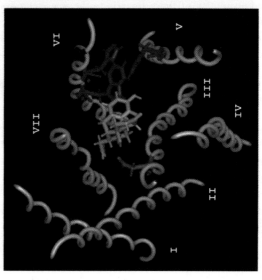

*Figure 4.5.   The docked structure of naloxone to the mu opioid receptor.  The cationic amine of the ligand (shown in yellow) is docked to the Asp of TM III with the phenolic moiety fills the aromatic pocket formed by TM V and VI (green).  These two receptor sites represent the opioid message recognized/displayed by all three receptor types.*

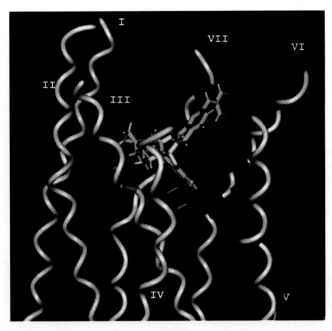

*Figure 4.6. The docked structure of GNTI to the kappa opioid receptor. The positively charged guanidinyl group of the ligand (shown in yellow) recognizes the kappa address Glu VI:23 (shown in blue).*

on the receptor, two positions, VI:23 and VII:03, can be shown to have direct interactions with the ligands. More importantly, these positions are variant among the mu, delta, and kappa types, suggesting a potential role in conferring selectivity for this ligand class. In kappa, VI:23 is a glutamate, while in delta and mu this position is occupied by tryptophan and lysine, respectively. Several site directed mutagenesis studies have now been reported that verify the role of Glu 297 (position VI:23) in determining the selectivity of norBNI and gNTI to the kappa receptor [82,83]. The most rational explanation for this site-specific function is the formation of a salt bridge from the cationic amine of the ligand to the carboxyl group of Glu 297. Further support for this hypothesis can be found in mutational studies of the delta receptor in which tryptophan VI:23 (W284 in the delta receptor numbering scheme) is replaced by a glutamate. This delta mutant shows an increased affinity for norBNI suggesting direct participation of glutamate VI:23 in ligand binding [83]. In delta, the pocket comprised of position VI:23 is more hydrophobic. Although not directly ver-ified with ligand binding studies, it has been hypothesized that tryptophan

VI:23 recognizes the indole moiety of NTI as well as other hydrophobic address components of related delta ligands. Unfortunately, a similar function has not been indicated for lysine VI:23 of the mu receptor. Attempts to design selectivity elements into NTI to take advantage of this positively charged site in the mu receptor have been unsuccessful raising some doubt as to the function of this residue in imparting mu-selectivity. The second site that has been linked with selectivity, VII:03, appears to function through a different mechanism. Mutational analysis of this position has shown a significant increase in the binding affinity of NTI at the mu and kappa receptors when the bulky aromatic sidechains that occupy VII:03 are replaced with alanine [83]. This suggests that tryptophan VII:03 in mu, and tyrosine VII:03 in kappa function to exclude delta selective ligands such as NTI by sterically hindering the putative address site.

NON-OPIATE LIGANDS

There are an ever-increasing number of non-opiate ligands that are designed to selectively bind to opioid receptors. Here, two well-studied examples are examined for comparison with the benzomorphinans. The final docked structure of the mu-selective agonist 3-methylfentanyl and the delta selective agonist SNC-80 [84]. (a representative diarylpiperazine) are shown in Figure 4.7a and 7b. Consistent with site directed mutagenesis studies [85,86], both ligands salt link through protonated amines with the conserved Asp in helix III. Methylfentanyl, however, adopts a unique orientation that places the N-phenethyl group deep into a crevice formed by helices II and III while the propanamide group projects upward towards TM helices III, VI, and VII. (For a complete description of automated docking and the binding site model, see ref [80].) Support for the model can be found in chimeric studies which suggest TM helices I-Ill and VI and VII are involved in sufenatnil binding [87] as well as comparitive studies with N-phenethylnormorphine. Molecular overlays of the opioid core of the docked naloxone structure in Figure 4.4 with N-phenethylnormorphine, and the independently docked 3-methylfentanyl indicate the phenethyl groups occupy the same putative binding pocket deep within the TM domain. A comparison of the docked structures is shown in *Figure 4.8*. It is also evident that fentanyl does not reach the "address" site at the TM-EL boundary near TM VI. This may explain the failure of site directed mutagenesis studies to pinpoint mu-selectivity sites in this TM boundary region. Moreover, the analysis indicates mu-selectivity may be conferred through a unique mechanism (as compared to the case of GNTI and NTI described above) involving a binding pocket formed by residues of TM helices II and III deep within the TM domain. It is important to point out that N-phenethylnormorphine is significantly more potent than morphine, lending support to this hypothesis.

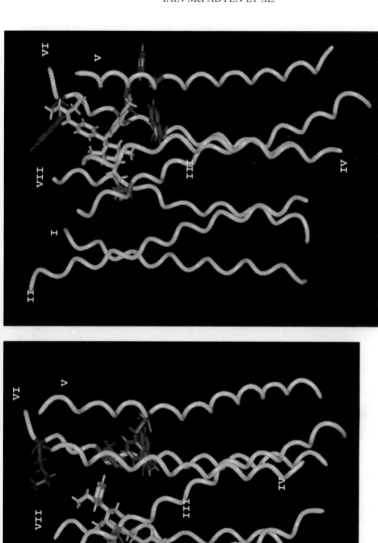

*Figure 4.7. Docked structures of methylfentanyl (A) and SNC80 (B) to the mu and delta opioid receptors. The phenethyl group of methylfentanyl projects deep into a crevice between TM II and III of the mu receptor. The binding site model of SNC80 is comparable to that of the opiates with the piperazine ring anchored to Asp 11:08, the methoxyphenyl ring oriented towards the aromatic cluster in TM V and VI, and the amide projected into the putative selectivity site at the top of TM VI and VII (Trp VI:03).*

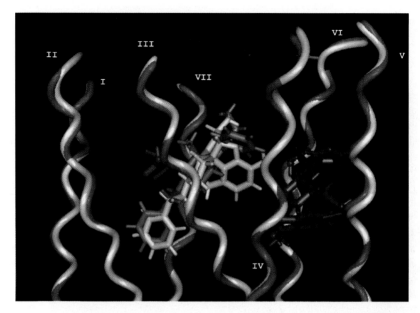

*Figure 4.8. Overlay of the receptor complexes of methylfentanyl (cyan) and N-phen-ethylnormorphine (yellow).*

The docking orientation of SNC-80 is somewhat comparable to that of the opiates. In previous structure-activity studies of substituted diarylpiperazines [88], it was suggested that the methoxyphenyl ring occupies the same pocket as the phenolic moiety of NTI, while the diethylamido-group projects into the putative delta-selectivity pocket at the TM boundary near helix VI. The docking orientation is supported by site directed mutagenesis studies which indicate the same delta-address site implicated in NTI binding (Trp VI:23), as well as two additional hydrophobic residues in EL-III (Val EL-III: 10 and Val EL-III: 11) are involved in high affinity binding of this class of compounds [89,90]. Although not routinely modeled in docking studies, EL-III is relatively short, placing these two valines in close proximity to tryptophan VI:23. These three residues may therefore form a hydrophobic pocket that is recognized by delta-selective ligands. Although not modeled here, it is important to add that N-phenethyl derivatives of the diarylpiperazines also have been reported and generally show increased muaffinity [88]. This lends further support to the existence of a unique mu-selectivity site and provides additional evidence to link different ligand classes through specific sites of recognition.

CONCLUSION

This chapter has described and applied methods to develop opioid GPCR structural models for use in molecular docking and drug design. Although the widespread cloning of GPCRs and the determination of high resolution X-ray data on rhodopsin has greatly advanced this field over the last decade, significant challenges still remain in the development of molecular models for predicting ligand binding and selectivity, function, and the structural basis to signal transduction. One of the greatest problems often encountered in building receptor models is structural refinement. It is becoming increasingly evident that GPCRs may adopt a variety of conformations across and within families. For example, a complete analysis of mutational data, biophysical studies, and ligand binding studies indicates that not all experiments can be rationalized based on one TM conformational model. In addition, it is difficult to explain the differences in selectivity and function noted for ligands within GPCR families using sequence information alone. Sequence identity within the TM domains of GPCR families can be high (e.g. the TM domains of delta, kappa, and mu opioid receptors). Small ligands such as fentanyl or arylacetamides (U50488) show few, if any, type-specific contacts, suggesting TM conformation may also play a role in determining selectivity [79,80]. Subtle differences in TM helix rotation, for instance, may alter the steric volume or surface of the cavity, yielding unique size-shape complementarities. Care must therefore be taken not to over-refine the tertiary structure of the TM domain using X-ray crystallographic data from structures like rhodopsin or bacteriorhodopsin. In terms of automated docking, refinement is critical since minor changes in the steric volume of the cavity can dramatically affect scoring. The models reported here are somewhat optimized in this regard and have been developed with a primary focus on ligand binding and recognition. To some extent, current models could be viewed as "averaged" structures since a wide range of data are accounted for in the model building. As more receptor-type specific data is available, however, these models will continue to evolve to capture individual conformational preferences for the receptors leading to more reliable automated docking and virtual screens.

Another limitation to the models reported here is the absence of loop structure and function in ligand binding and recognition. These structures are typically left off the TM domain in ligand binding studies since most evidence suggests small ligands, such as fentanyl, are bound within the TM domain cavity. This, however, is not true of peptides which clearly extend into the EL region. Previous studies have suggested potential functions of the loops in peptide binding and signal transduction but have fallen somewhat short of defining molecular conformations [91]. The great challenge in modeling the loops lies in the sequence variation displayed across GPCR families (as well as within families) and the lack of detailed information regarding specific binding sites or functions of the extracellular loops in ligand binding. While the molecular docking of relatively small ligands does not appear to require loop structures, an understanding of peptide recognition and perhaps insight into the mechanism of signal transduction lies in the determination of loop structure and function. In addition, the results presented above suggest that extracellular loop structures may form binding pockets at the TM-EL boundary, offering new targets for ligand design.

A very recent development in the GPCR field has been the identification of homo- and heterodimeric complexes of receptors, providing yet another challenge in model building receptor structures. First explored for muscarinic and adrenergic receptors [92], dimer structures have been reported for opioid receptors as well [93]. While the function of dimerization is not yet known, heterodimer formation may have a tremendous impact on ligand-mediated signal transduction. It is thought that dimers can either form a contact or interlocking pair. In the latter, the TM helices can domain swap producing a unique GPCR with modified pharmacology. A delta-kappa heterodimer, for example, could interlock and swap TM helices VI and VII, yielding a kappa-receptor that contains delta selectivity elements and a delta-receptor with kappa selectivity elements. (Note that TM helix VI contains a key site VI:23 involved in opiate selectivity.) A schematic of this dimer is shown in *Figure 4.9*. In this case, kappa-ligands could be agonists or antagonists of the delta-receptor, producing a very different pharmacological response than would be indicated by the monomeric model. Structurally, the receptors may adopt unique conformations as well, requiring a complete re-evaluation of the model building process. It is still not clear, however, if the opioid receptors form interlocking or simple contact dimers so attempts to account for domain swapping of the TM helices may be premature. In addition, ligand binding data strongly suggest that in most cases, the receptor-ligand complexes can be treated as monomers. Nevertheless, it will be interesting to explore the potential for allosteric regulation as well as modified selectivity through the concept of receptor dimerization. In fact, it may be possible to take advantage of dimeric structures in the development of new, bivalent ligands. Previous work has suggested that bi-

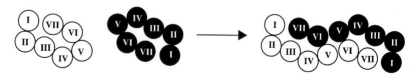

*Figure 4.9. Heterodimer formation showing potential domain swapping between receptors. In this model, selectivity elements from TM VI and VII are exchanged between receptors.*

valent ligands may be significantly more potent than their monovalent counterparts, offering new avenues for drug design and development [94].

One of the main applications of GPCR model building is the rationalization and development of structure-based concepts of ligand recognition. Here, we focused on the automated docking of naloxone and naltrexone-derived ligands. This well-studied group of ligands fit the classic message-address concept of recognition where the universal "message" or opioid core occupies the receptor cavity (which is well conserved in sequence identity across types) while the variable "address" site of the receptor (VI:23) recognizes the indole of NTI or the guanidinyl group of GNTI, for example. The success of automated docking in identifying correct docking orientations is not surprising given the amount, and success of site directed mutagenesis studies in locating potential sites of recognition. Shortly after the cloning of the opioid receptors, ligand binding studies identified three key sites of interaction for opiate-based ligands, including the highly conserved asp in TM III, a cluster of aromatic sidechains in TM V and VI, and a type-specific pocket at the TM VI-EL boundary (i.e. VI:23). There is little doubt that these results helped shape the structure of the TM domain over the years yielding a receptor model that works extremely well for opiates. For other ligand classes, the experimental results have not been as clear. While most studies suggest the conserved Asp in TM III is a key anchor for cationic amines of opioid ligands, attempts to unite opioid ligands through a common binding site model have, for the most part, failed. The binding affinity of small ligands, such as fentanyl or U50488 has not been shown to depend on aromatic residues in the pocket of the cavity. In addition, the selectivity of these ligands has not been linked with "addresses" associated with the opiates. One exception to this can be found in the binding of diarylpiperazines (SNC80). The binding affinity of this ligand class has been shown to depend on the delta-specific tryptophan at the top of TM VI (VI:23) and two valines in EL III. Although this suggests diarylpiperazines may also recognize the delta-address noted in opiate binding, it is important to point out that kappa-selective SNC80 analogs have not been reported. (Recall the relationship of NTI and GNTI to receptor selectivity.) It is therefore unclear at this point in time if "address" sites are universal or ligand specific. Moreover, each receptor type may display unique address elements as suggested by the apparent mu-affinity of N-phenethyl derivatives of morphine, diarylpiperazines, and fentanyl-based compounds.

In terms of ligand docking and virtual screening of non-opiates, the lack of experimental data, and the potential for multiple binding modes and sites, is problematic. While we have reported good success in identifying the most probable binding site models for a number of ligand classes, the application of automated docking protocols to virtual screening across ligand classes is far from straightforward. In most cases, a detailed analysis of the docking results, and comparisons with experimental ligand binding data, is required to interpret and assign significance to the DOCK scoring. Ligand flexibility adds yet another dimension to the docking problem. Although not discussed in detail here, past work on fentanyl and arylacetamides (U50488) has shown DOCK protocols must account for the potential for conformational variance in the ligand [79,80]. greatly increasing the size and complexity of the computational problem. Nevertheless, the results of automated docking (reported here and elsewhere) have yielded receptor-ligand complexes that are both predictive and informative in understanding the structural basis to binding and selectivity, especially if DOCK searches are conducted within ligand classes. While this suggests that virtual screening across diverse ligand databases may be out of the reach of current model resolutions, there is little doubt that the application will be expanded as more experimental and structural data on GPCRs becomes available and integrated into structural models of ligand-receptor recognition.

## REFERENCES

1   Dhawan, B. N., Cesselin, F., Raghubir, R., Reisine, T., Bradley, P. B., Portoghese, P. S., and Hamon, M. (1996) Pharmacol. Rev. 48, 567–592.

2   Childers, S. R. (1991) Life Sci. 48, 1991–2003.

3   Carter, B. D. and Medzihradsky, F. (1992) J. Neurochem. 58, 1611–1619.

4   Williams, J. T., North, R. A., and Tokimasa, T. (1988) J. Neurosci. 8, 4299–4306.

5   Seward, E. P., Hammond, C., and Henderson, G. (1991) Proc. R. Soc. Lond [Biol.] 244, 129–135.

6   Rang, H. P. and Dale, M. M. Pharmacology, Churchill Livingstone, Edinburgh (1987).

7   Aldrich J. V. Analgesics, in Burger's Medicinal Chemistry and Drug Discovery, ed. By Wolff, M. E., John Wiley & Sons, Inc., pp. 321–441, (1996).

8   Casy, A. F. and Parfitt, R. T. Opioid Analgesics: Chemistry and Receptors. Plenum Press, New York, (1986).

9   Collin E. (1999) Soins. 633, 15–18.

10  Martin, W. R., Eades, C. G., Thompson, J. A., Huppler, R. E., and Gilbert, P. E. (1976) J. Pharmacol. Exp. Ther. 197, 517–532.

11  Satoh, M. and Minami, M. (1995) Pharmacol. Ther. 68, 343–364.

12  Resine, T. (1995) Neuropharmacol. 34, 463–472.

13  Reisine, T. and Bell, G. I. (1993) Trends Neurosci. 16, 506–509.

14  Kieffer, B. L. (1995) Cellular and Molecular Neurobiol. 15, 615–635.

15  Baldwin, J. M., Schertler, G. F. X., and Unger, V. M. (1997) J. Mol. Biol. 272, 144–164.

16  Li, X., Keith, D. E., Jr., and Evans, C. J. (1996) FEBS Lett. 397, 25–29.

17  Darlison, M. G., Greten, F. R., Harvey, R. J., Kreienkamp, H. J., Stuhmer, T., Zwiers, H., Lederis, K., and Richter, D. (1997) Proc. Natl. Acad. Sci. U.S.A. 94, 8214–8219.

18  Barrallo, A., Gonzalez-Sarmiento, R., Porteros, A., Garcia-Isidoro, M., and Rodriguez, R. E. (1998) Biochem. Biophys. Res. Commun. 245, 544–548.

19  Zipser, B., Ruff, M. R., O'Neill, J. B., Smith, C. C., Higgins, W. J., and Pert, C. B. (1998) Brain Res. 463, 296–304.

20  Cadet, P. and Stefano, G. B. (1999) Mol. Brain Res. 74, 242–246.

21  Harrison, L. M., Kastin, A. J., Weber, J. T., Banks, W. A., Hurley, D. L., and Zadina, J. E. (1994) Peptides 15, 1309–1329.

22  Law, P. Y., Wong, Y. H., and Loh, H. H. (1999) Biopolymers 51, 440–455.

23  Schwartz, T. W. (1994) Curr. Opin. Biotechnol. 5, 434–444.

24  Gershengorn, M. C. and Osman, R. (2001) Endocrinol. 142, 2–10.

25  Bikker, J. A., Trumpp-Kallmeyer, S., and Humblet, C. (1998) J. Med. Chem. 41, 2911–2927.

26  Jones, D. and Thornton, J. M. (1993) J. Computer Aided Mol. Des. 7, 439–456.

27  Anthonsen, H. W., Baptista, A., Drablos, F., Martel, P., and Petersen, S. B. (1994) J. Biotechnol. 36, 185–220.

28  Bairoch, A. and Apweiler, R. (2000) Nucleic Acids Research 28, 45–48.

29  Berman, H. M., Westbrook, J., Feng, Z., Gilliland, G., Bhat, T. N., Weissig, H., Shindyalov, I. N., and Bourne, P. E. (2000) Nucleic Acids Research 28, 235–242.

30  Sali, A. (1995) Curr. Opin. Biotechnol 6, 437–451.

31  Chothia, C. and Leks, A. M. (1986) EMBO J. 5, 823–826.

32  Taylor, W. R. (1994) J. Biotechnol. 35, 281–291.

33  Kyte, J. and Doolittle, R. F. (1982) J. Mol. Biol. 154, 105–132.

34  Ballesteros, J. A. and Weinstein, H. (1995) Methods in Neurosci. 25, 366–428.

35  Donnelly, D., Overington, J. P., and Blundell, T. L. (1994) Protein Eng. 7, 645–653.

36  Samatey, F. A., Xu, C., and Popot, J.-L. (1995) Proc. Natl. Acad. Sci. U.S.A. 92, 4577–4581.

37  Richardson, J. S. and Richardson, D. C. (1988) Science 240, 1648–1652.

38  Presta, L. G. and Rose, G. D. (1988) Science 240, 1632–1641.

39  Muller, G. (2000) Curr. Med. Chem. 7, 861–888.

40  Luecke, H., Schobert, B., Richter, H.-T., Cartailler, J.-P., and Lanyi, J. K. (1999) J. Mol. Biol. 291, 899–911.

41  Palczewski, K., Kumasaka, T., Hori, T., Behnke, C. A., Motoshima, H., Fox, B. A., Le Trong, I., Teller, D. C., Okada, T., Stenkamp, R. E., Yamamoto, M., and Miyano, M. (2000) Science 289, 739–745.

42  Henderson, R., Baldwin, J. M., and Ceska, T. A. (1990) J. Mol. Biol. 213, 899–929.

43  Grigorieff, N., Ceska, T. A., Downing, K. H., Baldwin, J. M., and Henderson, R. (1996) J. Mol. Biol. 259, 393–421.

44  Donnelly, D., Findlay, J. B. C., and Blundell, T. L. (1994) Receptors & Channels 2, 61–78.

45  Baldwin, J. M. (1993) EMBO J. 12, 1693–1703.

46  Alkorta, I. and Loew, G. H. (1996) Protein Eng. 9, 573–583.

47  Papermaster, D. S. and Dreyer, W. J. (1974) Biochemistry 13, 2438–2444.

48  Schertler, G. F. X., Villa, C., and Henderson, R. (1993) Nature 362, 770–772.

49  Royant, A., Nollert, P., Edman, K., Neutze, R., Landau, E. M., Pebay-Peyroula, E., and Navarro, J. (2001) Proc. Natl. Acad. Sci. U.S.A. 98, 10131–10136.

50  Pogozheva, I. D., Lomize, A. L., and Mosberg, H. I. (1997) Biophysical J. 70, 1963–1985.

51  Pogozheva, I. D., Lomize, A. L., and Mosberg, H. I. (1998) Biophysical J. 75, 612–634.

52  Joseph-McCarthy, D. (1999) Pharmacol. and Ther. 84, 179–191.

53  Metzger, T. G., Paterlini, M. G., Portoghese, P. S., and Ferguson, D. M. (1996) Neurochem. Res. 21, 1287–94.

54  Jones, G. and Willett, P. (1995) Curr. Opin. Biotechnol. 6, 652–656.

55  Bissantz, C., Folkers, G., and Rognan, D. (2000) J. Med. Chem. 43, 4759–4767.

56  Ferrin, T. E., Huang, C. C., Jarvis, L. E., and Langridge, R. Midas Plus. (2.1). 2000. San Francisco, CA, Computer Graphics Laboratory, University of California.

57  Ferrin, T. E., Jarvis, L. E., and Langridge, R. (1988) J. Mol. Graphics 6, 13–27.

58  Pearlman, D. A., Case, D. A., Caldwell, J. W., Ross, W. S., Cheatham, III, T., Debolt, S., Ferguson, D. M., Siebel, G., and Kollman, P. A. (1995) Comp. Phys. Comm., 91, 1–41.

59  Cornell, W. D., Cieplak, P., Bayly, C. I., Gould, I. R., Merz, K. M. Jr., Ferguson, D. M., Spellmeyer, D. C., Fox, T., Caldwell, J. W., and Kollman, P. A. (1995) J. Am. Chem. Soc. 117, 5179–5197.

60  Meng, E. C., Shoichet, B. K., and Kuntz, I. D. (1992) J. Comput. Chem. 13, 505–524.

61  Connolly, M., Gschwend, D. A., Good, A. C., Oshiro, C., and Kuntz, I. D. DOCK, version 3.5. (3.5). 1995. San Francisco, CA, Department of Pharmaceutical Chemistry, University of California.

62  Alschul, S. F., Madden, T. L., Schaffer, A. A., Zhang, J., Zhang, Z., Miller, W., and Lipman, D. J. (1997) Nucleic Acid Res. 25, 3389-3402.

63  Thompson, J. D., Higgins, D. G., and Gibson, T. J. (1994) Nucleic Acid Res. 22, 4673–4680.

64  Rost, B., Casadio, R., Fariselli, P., and Sander, C. (1995) Prot. Sci. 4, 521–533.

65  Reithmeier, R. A. (1995) Curr. Opin. Struct. Biol. 5, 491–500.

66  Sankararamakrishnan, R. and Vishveshwara, 5. (1990) Biopolymers 30, 287–298.

67  Zhou, W., Flanagan, C., Ballesteros, J. A.; Konvicka, K. , Davidson, J. S., Weinstein, H., Millar, R. P. , Sealfon, S. C. (1994) Mol. Pharmacol. 45, 165–70.

68  Rao, V.R., Cohen, GB., Oprian, D.D. (1994) Nature, 367, 639–42

69  Nathans, J. (1990) Biochemistry, 29, 9746–52.

70  Fu, D., Ballesteros, J. A., Weinstein, H., Chen, J., Javitch, J. A. (1996) Biochemistry, 35, 111278–85

71  Javitch, J. A., Fu, D., Chen, J. (1995) Biochemistry, 34, 16433–39

72  Javitch, J. A., Ballesteros, J. A., Weinstein, H., Chen, J. (1998) Biochemistry, 37, 998–1006.

73  Dunbrack, R. L., Jr. (1999) Proteins: Structure, Function, Genetics, Suppl. 3, 81–87.

74  Dunbrack, R. L. Jr. and Karplus, M. (1993) J. Mol. Biol. 230, 543–574.

75  Laskowski, R. A., MacArthur, M. W., Moss, D. S., and Thornton, J. M. (1993) J. Appl. Cryst. 26, 283–291.

76  Frisch, M. J., Trucks, G. W., Schlegel, H. B., Gill, P. M. W., Johnson, B. G., Robb, M. A., Cheeseman, J. R., Keith, T., Petersson, G. A., Montgomery, J. A., Raghavachari, K., Al-Laham, M. A., Zakrewski, V. G., Ortiz, J. V., Foresman, J. B., Cioslowski, J., Stefanov, B. B., Nanayakkara, A., Challacombe, M., Peng, C. Y., Ayala, P. Y., Chen, W., Wong, M. W., Andres, J. L., Replogle, E. S., Gomperts, R., Martin, R. L., Fox, D. J., Binkley, J. S., Defrees, D. J., Baker, J., Stewart, J. J. P., Head-Gordon, M., Gonzalez, C., and Pople, J. A. Gaussian94, revision E2. 2001. Pittsburgh, PA, Gaussian Inc.

77  Cieplak, P., Cornell, W. D., Bayly, C. I., and Kollman, P. A. (1995) J. Comput. Chem. 16, 1357–1377.

78  Connelly, M. L. (1983) Science 221, 709–713.

79  Subramanian, G., Paterlini, M. G., Larson, D. L., Portoghese, P. 5., and Ferguson, D. M. (1998) J. Med. Chem. 41, 4777–4789.

80  Subramanian, G., Paterlini, M. G., Portoghese, P. S., and Ferguson, D. M. (2000) J. Med. Chem. 43, 381–391.

81  Takemori, A. E. and Portoghese, P. S. (1992) Annu. Rev. Pharmacol. 32, 239–69.

82  Jones, R. J., Hjorth, S. A., Schwartz, T. W., and Portoghese, P. S. (1998) J. Med. Chem. 41, 4911–4913.

83  Metzger, T. G., Paterlini, M. G., Ferguson, D. M., and Portoghese, P. 5. (2001) J. Med. Chem. 44, 857–862.

84  Calderon, S. N., Rothman, R. B., Porreca, F., Flippen-Anderson, J. L., McNutt, R. W., Xu, H., Smith, L. B., Bilsky, E. J., Davis, P., and Rice, K. C. (1994) J. Med. Chem. 37, 2125–2128.

85  Heerding, J., Raynor, K., Kong, H., Yu, L., and Reisine, T. (1994) Reg. Pept. 54, 119–120.

86  Befort, K., Tabbara, L., Bausch, S., Chavkin, C., Evans, C., and Kieffer, B. (1996) Mol. Pharmacol. 49, 216–223.

87  Zhu, J., Xue, J.-C., Law, P.-Y., Claude, P. A., Luo, L.-Y., Yin, J.-L., Chen, C.-G., and Liu-Chen, L.-Y. (1996) FEBS Lett. 384, 198–202.

88  Podlogar, B. L., Poda, G. I., Demeter, D. A., Zhang, S.-P., Carson, J. R., Neilson, L. A., Reitz, A. B., and Ferguson, D. M. (2000) Drug Design and Discovery 17, 34–50.

89  Valiquette, M., Vu, H. K., Yue, S. Y., Wahlestedt, C., and Walker, P. (1996) J. Biol. Chem. 271, 18789–96.

90  Li, X., Knapp, R. J., Stropova, D., Varga, E. V., Wang, Y., Malatynska, E., Calderon, S., Rice, K., Rothman, R., Porreca, F., Hruby, V. J., Roeske, W. R., and Yamamura, H. I. (1995) Analgesia 1, 539–42

91  Paterlini, M. G., Portoghese, P. S., and Ferguson, D. M. (1997) J. Med. Chem. 40, 3254–62.

92  Maggio, R., Vogel, Z., and Wess, J. (1993) Proc. Natl. Acad. Sci. U.S.A. 90, 3103–3 107.

93  Gomes, I., Jordan, J. A., Gupta, A., Trapaidze, N., Nagy, V., and Devi, L. A. (2000) J. Neurosci. 20, RC110(1–5).

94  Portoghese, P.S., Larson, D.L., Sayre, L.M., Yim, C.B., Ronsisvalle, G., Tam, S.W., and Takemori, A.E (1986) J. Med. Chem. 29, 1855–1861.

# Subject Index

# Cumulative Index of Authors for Volumes 1–40

*The volume number, (year of publication) and page number are given in that order.*

# Cumulative Index of Subjects for Volumes 1–40

*The volume number, (year of publication) and page number are given in that order.*

## DATE DUE